The Diet That Says "YES, YOU CAN!"

Yes, you can indulge in your favorite "no-no" foods without guilt

Yes, you can forget about every diet fad

Yes, you can personally design and completely control your own individual weight-loss program

Yes, you can defeat such poundage pitfalls as force-feeding friends and supermarket seductions

Yes, you can get the exercise you need without sweat or strain

Yes, you can finally succeed in breaking the "yo-yo" pattern of weight fluctuation and stay slim forever

Yes, you can join the many men and women who already have proven this radically new, permanent weight-loss method to be dramatically successful

EATING IS OKAY!

The book that tells you that you can do it!

Eating Is Okay!

*A Radical Approach
to Successful Weight Loss*

The Behavioral-Control Diet
Explained in Full

by
Henry A. Jordan, M.D.
Leonard S. Levitz, Ph.D.
Gordon M. Kimbrell, Ph.D.

Edited by Steve Gelman

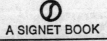

A SIGNET BOOK

NEW AMERICAN LIBRARY

COPYRIGHT © 1976 BY ASSOCIATES FOR BEHAVIORAL EDUCATION AND S. AND R. GELMAN ASSOCIATES, INC.

All rights reserved. For information address
Rawson Associates,
115 Fifth Avenue, New York, New York 10003.

This is an authorized reprint of a hardcover edition published by Rawson, Wade Publishers, Inc.
The hardcover edition was published simultaneously in Canada by McClelland an Stewart, Ltd.

SIGNET TRADEMARK REG. U.S. PAT. OFF. AND FOREIGN COUNTRIES
REGISTERED TRADEMARK—MARCA REGISTRADA
HECHO EN WINNIPEG, CANADA

SIGNET, SIGNET CLASSIC, MENTOR, ONYX, PLUME, MERIDIAN AND NAL BOOKS are published by NAL PENGUIN INC., 1633 Broadway, New York, New York 10019

FIRST SIGNET PRINTING, FEBRUARY, 1978

10   11   12   13   14   15   16   17   18

PRINTED IN CANADA

Dedicated

To

Barbara, Meryl, and Barbara

Contents

PART THREE   *Activity*

Acknowledgment

We wish to acknowledge the contribution of the many behavioral scientists whose work encouraged the formulation of a rational treatment for overweight people. We would also like to thank two long-time friends and colleagues who over the years have provided us with knowledge, support, and guidance, Dr. Eliot Stellar, Provost of the University of Pennsylvania, and Dr. Albert J. Stunkard, Professor of Psychiatry, Stanford University.

PART 1

How To
Begin

CHAPTER
1

The Start
of a New
Lifestyle

THE WOMAN LOOKED LIKE A LITTLE STUFFED TOY. SHE was five foot one and, when she came to us, 240 pounds. At the age of twenty-eight she lived with her father and brother. They were fat too.

She was motivated to lose weight; we determined that after only a few sessions at the weight-loss clinic we run at the University of Pennsylvania. And she had a good grasp of our philosophy—that in order to lose weight, and keep it off, you must make changes in your entire life-style. But it was difficult for her to change her life-style at home. No matter how many times she told her father and brother that she should no longer eat anywhere but at the table, they continued offering her endless extra food. Ice cream in the living room. Spaghetti on the patio. And one day apple pie—hot and steaming—in the den.

For seven weeks now she had been telling them,

imploring them, appealing to them. But they kept ignoring her. And here now, hot, luscious apple pie. What did she do? What could she do? She took the pie lovingly, put it down and, after a brief pause, stomped it to sauce with both feet.

The response was uncommonly dramatic. Everything else was patently symbolic—the impact of lifestyle, of family influence upon your weight; the importance of delivering and enforcing the message that "I must be in control of my own food intake and must assert myself in order to gain that control." And, indeed, although apple pie was the catalyst here, the main contention of our weight-loss method is that many factors, not merely food, contribute to fatness and cannot be controlled by traditional diet. When we speak of diet here, we do so exclusively in the context of its original Greek definition, "manner of living." Making changes in the way you live is the most critical goal of behavioral weight control.

SWITCHING TO AN ELECTRIC TYPEWRITER CAN MAKE YOU GAIN WEIGHT

The most important fact about weight loss is ridiculously simple: You take in calories through food, burn them up through activity, and gain weight when the caloric intake is greater than the caloric expenditure. It is a myth, then, that people get fat merely because they eat too much. The problem can be caused as much by shortage of physical activity as by overabundance of food. And not necessarily strenuous physical activity. It has been estimated, for example, that a typist who switches from a manual to an electric typewriter, and makes no other changes in lifestyle, will gain six pounds in one year.

The key—and this is nothing new—is achieving the balance of calories and activity to maintain weight or lose weight. Our innovation is to show how weight loss can be linked to every aspect of daily living. We do not tell you which foods to eat or not to eat. Rather, our methods and studies are rooted in human behavior. We discern, and this book will show, why people eat or do not; what our eating patterns tell us about ourselves; how age, sex, marital status, economic-social status, and family interactions strongly affect eating habits as well as weight. For a nation assaulted by endless diet books, for a country that spends $200 billion a year on food and more than 5 percent of that on reducing, we offer the particular view that individuals who change their life-styles are the ones, by and large, who will be successful in losing weight for a lifetime.

The changes can be small. Do you eat, without thinking, while talking on the telephone in the kitchen? Clearly you ought to make and take your calls in another room. Do you avoid climbing stairs? If you got in the habit of climbing stairs only five minutes a day, you could keep off more than ten pounds in two years.

We offer such suggestions and deeper ones, on an individual basis, to the patients who visit us one hour a week, for twenty weeks, at the Hospital of the University of Pennsylvania or at the Institute for Behavioral Education. Our Behavioral Weight-Control Program has been in operation for five years and is acknowledged as a pioneer in its field. Not long ago the *New York Times*, in an article on the many "serious scientific" methods of weight loss, judged that ours *"has had the most promising success to date in treating obesity,"* that *"to achieve permanent weight loss,"* a person *"must forever change those aspects of his behavior that made him fat in the first place."*

This book will show how you, as an individual, must take control of your own weight-loss program. It will show how you can analyze your habits to find out which ones contribute to overweight—and how you can change them. It will show how, gradually, over the long run of twenty weeks, you can not only lose from twenty to forty pounds, but can make enough substantive changes so that you will be unlikely to ever put back the weight you have lost. And beyond outlining a method for losing weight, it will help you understand the reasons you eat and get fat, and aid you in adjusting to a new image of yourself—and a new life.

WHY YOU'VE GAINED BACK WEIGHT IN THE PAST

Probably you have lost weight before. Maybe several times. Recently we received a letter from a woman who had raised a family, was now back in school, and had, over the course of her life, a history of substantial accomplishment. Her problem, she wrote, was that of continually losing weight and regaining it. Why, she wanted to know, was she motivated to do so many other things well but not to keep her weight down?

Her trouble, though, was not lack of motivation. Quite the opposite. People who continually lose weight are very highly motivated—or they wouldn't keep trying. But they have been snipping the weeds, not ripping out the roots. A hospital starvation program, say, will produce weight loss. So will a diet that tells you exactly what to eat, how much to eat, and when to eat. So will medically supervised drug therapies. Or a rigid limit of calories per day. Or—sometimes—gimmicky weight-loss programs. But nothing in any of these cases is being done to change the behavior that "made you fat in the first place." Suppose someone loses thirty pounds that he originally put on because he enacted most of his business deals at luncheons and dinners. How can he possibly maintain that weight loss if he doesn't understand the impact of his job on his weight and make appropriate adjustments?

Weight-loss programs rarely set any course at all for the future. They work while you are following strict guidelines, while you are putting responsibility for your weight loss on outer influences. You are likely to later take the attitude that, "Well, I'm just a poor soul wandering around, and the food's there, and I eat it, and I get upset that I ate it." And the product of all this, unfortunately, can be guilt.

People ask us at the beginning of treatment if there will ever be a time when they won't be so susceptible to food, if they'll ever be able to go into a bakery, buy a loaf of bread and look at the brownies and not even want them? We must answer: Probably not. Probably your taste for brownies won't change. But your way of handling it will.

You will, for starters, be in control of your own weight maintenance, and as part of that control, you will not be intimidated by your desire for a brownie or distraught if you decide to eat one. Indeed, one of our critical goals is to eliminate guilt. Particularly the guilt that can come with eating certain foods. It is a myth that you can lose weight or maintain weight loss only by saying no to your favorite foods. A thin person can eat a slice of fudge cake and enjoy it, period. A fat person eats the cake, feels guilty, worries, feels worse, and has a second slice, hopefully to boost his spirits. Eating develops into a moral issue, and that's ridiculous. Weight loss shouldn't be some kind of character-building experience in which you have to engage in a constant battle with your conscience. We try to emphasize the vital difference between will power and self-control. Will power is sitting in an ice-cream parlor and ordering coffee with artificial sweetener when you really want ice cream. We prefer *self-control. Have your dish of ice cream, but pass up dessert at dinnertime* to compensate for the calories. Or perhaps engage in some extra physical activity to burn them up.

Indeed, it is our contention that you ought to eat any kind of food you like. Milk shakes are okay. And pizza. And pasta. With proper planning. And moderation. Better to have 100 calories of candy—and be satisfied—than to eat the equivalent calories in a carload of celery and feel unsatisfied. One girl, who'd been in our program awhile, wanted an ice-cream cone so badly one night that she persuaded her father to drive eight miles for it. She took three bites of the cone, said she'd had enough, and listened raptly as her father computed the mileage—two and two-thirds miles per bite—at the top of his lungs. "But," she said, bless her, "they were the best three bites of ice cream I've ever had in my life."

That girl felt no need to gorge herself with ice cream; she knew she could have it regularly. Too often, though, if you're overweight, you're preoccupied with totally depriving yourself of a particular food. Then, if you eat it, your attitude is: "I've failed again. I'm no good. I'm not worth all the effort that it takes to try to lose weight, what's the use of it?" And the diet's generally over, at least for a while.

Will power? Morality in eating? Ridiculous. Why should fat people, without proper training, be expected to control their eating in situations where everybody else eats? And yet, they've been led to believe that it's a simple matter of will power. The society has said, "Look, fat person, don't eat so much! Learn to control yourself!" But what am I supposed to control against? And where are the mechanisms?

We provide the mechanisms, the training. We show how, throughout your life, food has been talking to you. And how you can now turn that around, how you can talk to the food.

Food? Talk? Indeed. You go to a restaurant, have your dinner, decide to decline dessert, and then the waiter wheels over the dessert cart. The probability of your having some pastry has appreciably risen because the food is right next to your chair, communicating with you. Or you go to a supermarket and the food is in an attractive package, perhaps a see-through package, and that food is sending out a message: "Buy me. Take me home." Or you arrive at a cocktail party, and a spread is laid out—beautiful, sumptuous—and the hostess or waitress is directing you to it.

You're at a dinner party at the home of a good friend. She's spent all day in the kitchen cooking, and people are saying, "This is a fantastic meal. You must have spent hours doing this!" And when the hostess says, "Yes, these are new recipes I just found," you feel almost morally obligated to please her and eat more food. She says, "Would you like some seconds?" And you feel you're going to hurt her feelings if you refuse.

There are ways in which you can exert control in

such situations, ways in which you can take charge of your own eating behavior, your own weight loss, and, later, your own weight maintenance.

First, you must be ready to face up to the responsibility. And the facts. One woman who came to our clinic had the habit of eating two dinners. At six o'clock she'd eat with her son, who would then leave for night school. At eight, when her husband came home from work, she'd have dinner with him. Neither the husband nor son knew she was eating with the other. And the woman herself felt that what was important was the appearance she gave other people. By eating a little with each, she gave them the impression she was not gorging herself.

In another home, there was no blunt acknowledgment, ever, of the state of the mother's body. In fact, she would not allow anyone to even use the word "fat" in the house. Until her three-year-old daughter brought everyone to their senses by asking, one day: "Would you please cut the heavy off my meat?"

No more rationalizing. We know of one woman who insisted she always had a light breakfast. When asked for the menu, she listed an egg, bacon or sausage, coffee, four pieces of toast. "Now there," she was told, "you see? There is a place where you could cut down on calories without making a big sacrifice. Why not have just one slice of toast instead of four?"

She was indignant. "But it's a four-slice toaster!"

Absurd? Of course. Absolutely absurd. But it happened. And the point is that, at the core, how much more absurd was her view than yours when you feel obligated to eat the whole pizza just because you ordered it?

Indeed, it is easy to laugh at someone shifting responsibility from herself onto an amalgam of metal and hot electric coils. But have you ever said, perhaps with your own personal variation:

"I wasn't hungry, but Aunt Sophie cooked my favorite food just for me. I couldn't hurt her feelings by refusing to eat a lot."

"The only reason I bought the doughnuts was so that I would have something for the kids to eat after school. You know how starved they are."

"I got mad at him. Before I knew it, I had eaten the whole pan of fudge. Why does he treat me like that?"

"The restaurant serves too much food. Is that my fault? It's a sin to waste food."

"I was going out to dinner with my new boyfriend and I didn't want him to think I was a glutton. So I ate a few sandwiches before going."

"Bob likes to have snacks while watching TV. If he wouldn't eat them, I wouldn't either."

"I don't have time to get more exercise. I have to be at work at nine."

"What else is there to do when you are lonely except eat?"

We have heard all these rationalizations, and thousands more, at our clinic. And we have been able to provide means for coping. There are many reasons why you may be fat; perhaps it is even a biological problem. But no matter the cause of your obesity, you can, with the proper mix of activity and conscious eating behavior, lose weight. Just because you may be biologically different doesn't mean that you can't control your body size. And that's the whole message: Anyone can lose.

Except. Except if your own medical doctor tells you not to try to lose weight. We do not accept patients at our clinic until we receive a report from their doctors listing, among other information, pertinent medical history (including diabetes, hypertension, gout, and pulmonary, hyperlipedimia, cardiovascular, neurological history), plus current medication, blood-pressure reading, laboratory studies on fasting blood sugar, cholesterol, triglycerides. We require each patient to have a medical examination before undertaking our program. We urge you to do the same. And be absolutely certain to specifically ask your physician:

1. "Is there any reason why I should not lose weight?"

2. "Is there any reason why I cannot engage in mild to moderate exercise?"

3. "Are there any restrictions on the type of food that I can eat?"

BREAKING THE HABITS OF A LIFETIME

We want you to eliminate habits that have contributed to your obesity and replace them with habits more suitable to your current goal of weight loss and your eventual goal of weight maintenance. If a man from Mars came to Philadelphia and someone stuck a gun in his face, he might not react at all; perhaps in his culture there are no guns. If that happened to any of us, we'd be terrified; we've learned to be afraid of guns. Our reactions to food also have been learned—and, with effort, can be changed. So can our reactions to situations that currently produce a need in us for food.

Breaking a habit, of course, is not easy. It may be deeply embedded. We had one patient who kept cookies in a kitchen drawer. Whenever she stood near the back door talking to her neighbor, she would automatically open the drawer and eat cookies. Finally, she removed all cookies from the drawer. But for a long time after that she'd stand talking at the back door and dip into the empty drawer, reaching for cookies.

Our program is a compilation of small, easily manageable steps, which ultimately add up to a very substantial life-style change. And the first small steps we suggest are behavior changes that will offer you a feeling of immediate accomplishment and, equally important, help set a pattern for the future.

You will have to learn to assert yourself. So, for a start, we want to direct your attention to everyday situations that you accept simply because you're reluctant to speak up. Are there times when you don't want to eat bread, don't want it near you in the restaurant, but feel you'll be bothering the waiter if you ask him to remove it—and you end up eating it? Convince yourself that his job is to serve you. At least once this week, if you're eating out, ask for some special accommodation from the waiter. Ask for a glass of water. Or for the entree to be served without potatoes. Or ask him to take the rolls off the table.

The idea of physical activity may seem at the start too jarring, but you could try one simple little thing. Park your car two hundred yards from your destination, rather than right beside it. Or, if you take a bus, get off one stop sooner—that's just two blocks in most cities. By walking briskly just eight hundred yards a day—two round trips to and from your car—you can burn off roughly five pounds in a year.

At the table start leaving a little food on your dish, even a teaspoonful at first, until you learn that your stomach, not an empty plate, ought to offer the signal to stop eating. And, most critically, slow down the pace of your eating. Slowing down will enable you to savor your food—and one of your ultimate goals is *to eat less, but enjoy it more.* Slowing down will immediately cut down the amount you eat because—and we've done laboratory experiments that prove this— for some reason the stomach takes awhile to signal you after it's full. Surely you've experienced a time when you've been very, very hungry and, after attacking the food rapidly, you say, "Wow, I finally had enough." And you stop. And then ten minutes later you say, "Wow, I really ate too darn much." If you eat very slowly, you'll get the signal before you overeat.

There are several ways you can slow down your eating. Swallow the food in your mouth before you load up the fork again. Or before you cut any more. Pick out someone in the room who may be eating slower than you and fall in with that person's pace. Put the fork down between bites. Put the sandwich down. Use the table napkin frequently. Chew thoroughly and slowly. Pay attention to the taste. Take sips of noncaloric beverage between bites; this not only slows down eating, but adds volume to the stomach, helping to fill you up.

And stick to it, even in the face of odd circumstances. One patient of ours had made many changes in her eating behavior. She had learned to leave food on her plate. She had learned to slow down her eating. She had learned to sip water to help her fill up. Now she was seated in a restaurant waiting for the meal and, rather than eating rolls, she was drinking a lot of water. A woman at the next table, a total stranger, walked over. "Why are you drinking all that water?" The patient began to stammer an answer, but the stranger cut back in, "You're going to ruin your appetite," and returned to her own meal.

Soon, the order came, and our friend began eating. She ate very, very slowly, as she had taught herself to do. She took sips of water between bites. The stranger kept staring and then, abruptly said, "How come you're eating so slowly? Aren't you ashamed of yourself? People are waiting for tables, everybody else is eating fast, and you're sitting here eating so slowly."

Our friend had made many adjustments for her new life. But she had never come up against anything—or anyone—like this. "Look," she finally said, "I'm sitting here enjoying my food. The only way for me to enjoy my food is to eat very slowly and relish each bite." And, again, the stranger subsided.

Everyone at our friend's table finished eating. Except her. When she finally stopped, there was food left over on her plate. Whereupon the stranger was at her again: "See, I told you if you drank that water . . ."

Most of the time, though, we learn of slightly different reactions to our patients' new habits. We heard recently of a woman who, in her own words, "was invited to a party where I tried very hard not to overeat. For hors d'oeuvres I had cauliflower and carrots. At the buffet I took a small piece of chicken and a teaspoonful of rice and a large salad, then I sat down at the dining-room table and had a good time and didn't eat any rolls.

"Finally the hostess cleared away everything, then brought in ten immense chocolate mousses with bittersweet chocolate inside and a whole cupful of whipped cream on each one. There was mine, sitting in front of me—and I panicked. I started watching the people around me, and eight of the ten people at the table just dug in and ate the whole chocolate mousse, attacking it so thoroughly with the spoon that the glass looked like it had come out of a dishwasher. There wasn't a speck left. And I did the same thing with mine.

"But there was one person left. The woman opposite me. I started watching her. She ate about half of it at a normal rate, and then she started pushing it around and picking up a spoonful and getting it halfway to her mouth and then putting it down again and then bringing it up again and talking to the person on her left and talking to me and putting it down again. And it was driving me crazy. So I said to her, 'May I ask you a question?' And she said, 'What?' And I said, 'I've been very interested in the way you're eating that chocolate mousse. Would you tell me—this is a multiple-choice question—(a) Are you allergic to chocolate? Or (b) do you dislike chocolate? Or (c) did you decide ahead of time to eat half of it for weight reasons? Or (d) could you not eat another spoonful? Or (e) none of the above?'

"She said, 'I couldn't eat another spoonful.' And I said, 'I never heard of such a thing.' And she said, 'I just completed the behavioral weight-control program at Penn.' And I said, 'Give me the telephone number.' And that's why I'm calling you now: to enroll."

PART 2

Food

CHAPTER
2

Why Do
You Eat?

DOES A POTATO-CHIP COMMERCIAL SPEED YOU TO THE cupboard? Is a midnight snack a family ritual? Do you automatically reach for nuts when they are poured into a living-room bowl? Or step without thinking to the popcorn counter at the movies? Probably you do. And you are eating, practically each and every such time, for reasons unrelated to hunger.

There are, indeed, myriad reasons why people eat—the least of which is hunger. And a fat person is no different in this regard from a thin one. But where a person of "normal" weight can routinely have a midnight snack and eat nuts in front of the TV or popcorn at the movies, these are usually unwise indulgences for a person trying to lose weight. It is important, then, if you want to reduce, to find out why you eat, to understand the forces driving you toward food. The ultimate aim is to get you in the habit of asking—and answering—a single question: "Why am I

in this place at this particular time with this food in
my hand, about to eat it?"

The more you understand, the better equipped you
are to cope. And it is important to understand, in tan-
dem with the reasons why you eat, that you very
likely have misconceptions about fat people in general. It is a myth, for example, that they eat more
food than others. Or eat more often. Or eat alone
more. Our studies show that many fat people do eat a
lot, and often, and alone. But so do an approximately
equal number of people of normal weight.

Have you been told, perhaps, that fat people snack
more than others? Not so, according to our findings at
the university. Or eat faster? Not so, either. In fact,
when we observed clientele in fast-food franchises, it
was a rather tiny fellow who set the speed record in
the Big Mac/Whopper/Super Shef category. Four-
teen seconds. Three bites.

Probably you have a misconception of your own
problem. Six out of seven people who come to us
describe themselves as compulsive eaters. And they
are wrong. Others insist they'll never lose weight until
they learn to say no to their favorite foods. And they,
most emphatically, are wrong. Still others say the
trouble is that they "go on binges."

Binge? What's a binge?

"Well, I sat down and ate half a cake."

That's not a binge. On a binge you feel something
has happened to you, that you're going to lose control. And then you start eating indiscriminately.
Maybe you'll go to three or four different restaurants
and eat full-course meals, one right after the other,
staggeringly large amounts of food. Most people who
tell us they've been on binges are simply feeling
guilty because of eating a little extra food some night.

It is a myth that overweight people have less will

power than others. Or that some people can never lose weight because of glandular imbalance. There are biological influences that make it tough for some people to lose weight and tough for others to fatten up. But, again, anyone can alter his or her weight.

Finally, it is a myth that people get fat because they are emotional messes. Every study we know about has proven there is no deep-rooted psychological problem that would produce the need to get fat. Overweight people do eat in response to stress. But so do underweight people. And all could just as easily have gotten into the habit of doing something else to alleviate anxiety.

One patient of ours was still angry hours after a morning argument with his family. So he didn't go straight home from work. He went to a bar, had some drinks, then to a restaurant, had a big dinner, and finally to the movies, where he ate a big box of popcorn. Then he went home, feeling fine. Probably he could have reduced his anger a better way. If your credit card gets messed up in the computer, your first reaction shouldn't be to eat. First, try to deal with the computer people. If you can't, try to find something other than food to ease your emotions.

A woman at our clinic realized that she always seemed to eat upon returning home from a visit to her mother. The reason, she figured out, was anxiety at the prospect of having to put the mother in a nursing home. Well, if you have, say, marital problems, you don't have to get a divorce in order to be thin. But you must learn that food is not going to solve the problem, even though it temporarily makes you feel good.

Of course, food is one of the first tranquilizers you ever encounter. As an infant you are fed when you cry. And as a child you are calmed with sweets when-

ever you bump your head, bruise your knee, or even
have your feelings hurt.

HOW YOUR FAMILY BACKGROUND
INFLUENCES YOUR EATING TODAY

If your childhood experiences at the dinner table
were unpleasant—because of arguments, perhaps, or
discipline—you may tend to snack a great deal today;
your pleasurable eating, see, took place between
meals. Or you may snack a lot because your family
didn't eat together very often or didn't pay much attention to food at meals. And because meals were
rushed in your home, you may now be having some
trouble slowing down the pace of your eating.

Are you having trouble following our advice to
leave a little food on your plate? Probably because of
your mother's pleadings in behalf of starving children
somewhere. But when your parents told you to "clean
your plate," and then bestowed rewards, you were
little and they were big and you needed their love.
Why persist now?

We've rarely heard of a mother who blames herself,
deep down, for a child's obesity. Rather, the attitude
is: "Gee, you're too fat—but here, eat all these things
I'm fixing for you." The reasoning, we suppose, is: "If
you would just eat what I fix, then you would be
okay. You're doing a lot of snacking and garbage
eating on the outside. That's why you're fat. Your
mother is not making you fat. She's fixing you nice,
wholesome food. If you'd just eat that, then you
would be okay."

One of us once observed an overweight family at a
diner. The mother, father, and teen-age son were gob-

bling double burgers and French fries. The daughter, who appeared to be about eight, abruptly put down her spoon, leaving ice cream in her sundae dish. "What's wrong?" said the mother.

"I don't want any more," said the girl. "I'm full."

"Full?" said the mother. "Are your arms full? Are your legs full? Eat! Don't be wasteful."

That girl will always struggle against fat because her mother has separated eating from all the normal internal signals of hunger. The girl will grow up fearing hunger, equating it with a sense of emptiness and a lack of well-being.

Some people who come to our clinic say they are never hungry. Never. When they then lose some weight and begin experiencing emptiness in the stomach, or gnawing, they can get a little surprised, occasionally fearful. We sometimes tell them: "Look at it this way. Think of the very time you're feeling hungry as the very time you're drawing upon your fat stores and actually losing weight." Some people say: "Do you have any good evidence of that?" And we say: "No, it's just an idea, but it may help make at least mild degrees of hunger a more pleasant experience."

Some people are moved by the first twinge of hunger: "Okay, let's stop and get something to eat." Others eat in anticipation of hunger: "Yes, I know I just ate lunch an hour ago, but I won't get another chance to eat until seven o'clock, so I'd better get something now." We often tell people that if they would learn to eat only when they are hungry, many of their weight problems would be solved.

Biologically, we need to eat to stay alive. But our biological makeup imposes other influences on our eating too. The aroma of food can produce salivation, a biological response. And our craving for sugar has biological roots. It has been proven that even in the first day of life an infant will prefer sugar water to plain unflavored water, and the food industry has capitalized on this. In the United States today each of us consumes on an average 102 pounds of sugar per year. For the food industry sugar serves as a cheap source of carbohydrates, as a good preservative, and as an appetite stimulant. Because it's so highly palatable, people will tend to eat more of a sugared food than the body may really require. And when that happens, you are eating because of anticipated taste, because signals from your mouth and palate are overwhelming those from lower down. Consider, for example, how many times you've heard someone say: "I'm full. I don't have room for another bite." And quickly correct himself: "But I'll make room for dessert."

A craving, an anticipated taste—anything giving out a signal that eating would be a good thing to do—is known as a food cue. The potato-chip commercial on TV is a food cue. The presence of food—that bowl of nuts in the living room—is a cue. The popcorn counter in the movies has become, because of habit, a cue. Even the time of day—"Oops, almost missed lunch"—can be a food cue.

As a cue for children the supermarket stocks certain foods on the lower shelves, at their eye level. Manufacturers put artificial coloring in food to make it more appealing to your eye. They package food in see-through plastic so you will be attracted by the sight. They finance advertising that not only tells you a food is delicious, but links the eating of it with happy occasions, even sometimes suggests it will help you attract the opposite sex.

Food cues clearly influence eating. We did a study once in a cafeteria, leaving the top of the ice cream freezer open one day and closed the next. With the top open, ice cream constituted 17 percent of the desserts selected by fat people and 16 percent of the desserts selected by others. When the ice cream was not clearly visible, it accounted for only 3 percent of the desserts eaten by obese people and only 5 percent of those taken by others.

SOCIAL PRESSURES THAT CAN MAKE YOU FAT

Because of modern technology and affluence America is progressively assaulted by an increase in food cues. This is the best-packaged country in the world. The availability of food is tremendous. On every neon strip in the nation fast-food franchises implore you to eat even if you are in a hurry, *particularly* if you're in a hurry. In markets everywhere you can buy packages of bread, cake, cooked macaroni—anything—to be kept at home ready to eat at any time. Many people have freezers. Today ice cream can be stored, whereas not all that long ago it just couldn't be available all the time.

Americans have grown accustomed to stocking their homes with convenience foods—foods that are easy to prepare, foods that are highly palatable. Our affluence, linked to our biological cravings for such foods, has made us vulnerable—as a whole society—to overeating. The food industry knows that if you want a particular food at ten o'clock at night, you're unlikely to go out shopping. So it encourages you to store the food in the house. And whereas a century ago, if you wanted a certain kind of late snack, you had to go to your root cellar or down to your spring house in the dark, there's no effort needed now. You have a refrigerator. You have a freezer. And possibly you even own that newest abomination for weight-conscious people, a microwave oven. Today if you're considering whether or not to eat a frozen food, you don't even have the dilemma: "Do I want to put it in the stove and wait half an hour for it?" You can have it out of your microwave oven in two minutes.

Even with segments of the population literally in danger of starving to death, there is more food available in the United States than ever before. And less expenditure of energy. Not long ago a new product was placed on the market, a grill for preparing breakfast or snacks at your bedside. So you could get food and zero physical activity simultaneously.

You eat because food is available. You eat out of frustration. You eat to be sociable. In low-income families, particularly, food sits at the center of social activities; while eighty-three cents is a lot of money for a bag of cookies, it is nevertheless a manageable amount, whereas ten dollars to take a family to the movies is not.

You eat to unwind. A drink or a snack marks the transition from the day at the job to the evening at home.

You eat out of boredom. People stock their cars with food to break the monotony of a long drive.

You eat because of tradition. Three meals a day is a habit, not a need an infant is born with.

You eat because society regards it as a priority. That is, if you are a housewife with a million things to do, you won't let yourself take time out for a relaxing twenty minutes in a bubble bath. But if you tell yourself you're hungry, that licenses you, in this society, to sit down and eat. At work you can't simply take a break to stroll around the building; people will look at you oddly and you'll feel you are not being productive. But you can go into the coffee room and sit down with a doughnut and coffee. And if you're a student, you often eat not so much out of hunger, but out of need for a study break. Who's going to deny a hungry person food?

A person living alone, with few interests and few friends, is liable to eat more from boredom than any other reason. A person with problems on the job may eat out of frustration. Someone bound down suddenly to a house and a new baby may eat more than ever for both reasons, boredom and frustration.

Someone starting to date or particularly interested in finding a spouse may tend to eat less than at any other time in life. So might someone just out of college and new to a job, full of hustle and often skipping meals. But at forty any of these same people may be in plumply comfortable ruts at home and may have earned fattening expense accounts at work.

When we get patients together in groups at the clinic, we regularly discuss the reasons people eat. And our patients often blurt out, in reaction to one another's stories: "That's the way it is with me too. That's where I fit in." Probably that has happened to you here. Our next step, then, is to show you how to solve your problem.

CHAPTER
3

Taking Charge
of Your Own
Weight Loss

SHE HAD A SOFT VOICE, A BUOYANT SMILE, AND WAS UN-
questionably one of the sweetest girls we'd ever met.
And sadly, the least assertive. On her job she constantly worked overtime without pay. At home her
family continually made demands upon her free time.
Three or four days a week, even when she had plans,
her parents or married brother would ask her to
baby-sit. She never said no.

Once, typically, she was all dressed up to go out
and a sister suddenly asked to be driven to the airport. "And," said the sister, "we've got to pick up my
friends too."

It was raining. And our patient was late for a date.
And the request could have been made weeks earlier,
when the sister and friends were planning the vacation. But no matter. She drove them to the airport.
She got them there on time. She even, when asked,

carried much of their luggage from the car to the check-in counter.

Her weight? How did all this affect her weight? Variously. She was unable to assert herself at home or elsewhere in regard to food. What's more, each time someone made a demand upon her, she would accede pleasantly. But inside she boiled. Angry. Frustrated. Depressed. And she made herself feel better by eating.

Another patient had learned quickly how vulnerable she was to food cues. She was working hard, therefore, to limit the availability of food at home and, since she lived alone, wasn't having much trouble. One day, though, she went to a wedding, declined dessert, and upon returning home, opened the refrigerator—and saw a big hunk of the wedding cake.

Her mother had been at the wedding too. And had seen her pass up the cake. She had thought that, really, her daughter deserved some delicious wedding cake. Our patient had already made it clear that she, and she alone, was going to control her food intake. So the mother didn't argue. Instead, she left early, came to the daughter's home, let herself in, and deposited the cake.

And our patient ate it.

This next patient worked the night shift. She would get home at about 7:30 A.M. each morning and sit around, waiting for her husband to awake. While waiting, she would eat. Then at 8:30 she would keep him company at breakfast and eat some more.

She did not really want all that food. But she did want to see her husband before he left for work. And she was bored waiting for him to awake. Once he was up, she wanted them to share some moments and activity, but all he had time for was breakfast.

She couldn't break the habit—until the morning she arrived home, went straight to the bed, shook him, and said, "Get out of bed. I want to dance."

He looked at her oddly. He was convinced she was out of her mind. But he got up. And danced.

The contrast is clear. While the first patient did not yet have the slightest control of her life, the second had made a good start; ideally, though, she should have simply thrown the cake away and not felt that the fates were giving her license to eat it. The third, meanwhile, not only was taking command of her own behavior, but was signaling her husband that he—as well as she—would have to make concessions to their mutual needs.

We are not suggesting bloody dispute. Not at all. It was unfortunate, we think, that a delicatessen clerk said to one of our patients: "How come someone as fat as you is buying potato salad?" And that she shot back: "You don't tell me whether to diet or not and I won't tell you whether to get a nose job or not."

But we do urge you to take charge of your own weight loss. You must. If you shift responsibility to friends or family, it can lead to, among other things, "sneak eating." One woman asked her teen-age daughters to reprimand her whenever they caught her eating something fattening; as a result, instead of sitting down in the open with, say, two chocolate chip cookies, she'd gobble down six on the sly. Another patient put her husband in charge of food shopping and storage and asked him to bawl her out whenever he spotted a slice or two of bread missing. He would literally count slices before leaving for work, but she soon found out how to fool him: by finishing up a whole loaf and then buying a replacement.

At the clinic we want to know if you're losing weight to please us, the doctors. If so, you're setting yourself up in a dependency relationship; whenever anything goes wrong, you'll be able to shift blame: *Come up with something new, doctor. Make me do something. Solve my problem for me.* Our method requires twenty-four-hour-a-day responsibility. Yours.

Set your own goals. And aim for gradual weight loss. If you've got a lot to lose, you may feel discouraged at setting a slow pace. Most of our patients feel that way. But after a while they invariably say, "Hey, this is not as hard as I thought it would be. I'm going about life having a good time, eating foods I like, and I'm getting a couple of pounds lighter every week."

View your weight loss as a progression of small accomplishments. Think in terms of five-pound or ten-pound units. And work them off at the rate of a few pounds a week.

THE FIRST STEPS

Your first step now is to make behavior changes geared to reducing the number of calories you consume. How many calories should you eat a day? That depends. On you. Figure it out on your own. To maintain weight, *for each pound you weigh, eat 10 calories a day if you get little physical activity, 14 a day if you are active.* If you weigh 160 pounds, then, and are moderately active, you ought to be able to maintain your weight on—160 multiplied by 12—1,920 calories a day, or 13,440 a week. This is a very rough guess.

It takes 3,500 calories to produce a pound of fat.

When the body does not get enough calories to maintain its weight, it draws on fat stores for energy. If you deprive the body of 3,500 calories needed for maintenance, therefore, it draws away one pound of your fat reserves. So, if you maintain your weight on 13,440 calories a week, you should lose one pound in a week by cutting back 3,500 calories, limiting yourself to 1,420 calories a day, or 9,940 over the week.

There are slight variations, depending on the individual; you may be more active, or less, than you think. So you must figure out your own calorie limit, stick to it for a couple of weeks, and check the results. You may find that you don't lose weight at 1,420 calories a day, but do at 1,350. Experiment. And remember that after you lose weight, even a little, you have established a new, lower maintenance level. So in order to continue losing weight, you'll have to lower your calorie intake still further. Or increase your physical activity.

The idea of increasing physical activity is important. Suppose that right now you weigh 130 pounds, or less, and want to lose weight. If you get mild physical activity, are 130, and apply our formula—130 multiplied by 12—you will maintain your weight at 10,920 calories a week. To lose two pounds in a week, you will have to cut down to 3,920 calories, an average of 560 a day. To lose 1½ pounds, you can eat only 5,670 calories a week, or 810 a day. But at 560 your health might be in danger, and at 810 you might feel deprived and have trouble sticking to your weight-loss program. It is better, if you are in these lower weight ranges, to plan on losing at the rate of, say, one pound a week, and to do so by increasing your physical activity as well as rationing your calories. For example, to lose half-a-pound through activity, all you have to do is burn up 1,750 more calories a week than you are doing now. This could be accomplished by a moderate amount of walking each day, or by any number of other ways we will describe later on.

You may have counted calories before, in other programs. But don't fall into the trap of taking a traditional approach now. Don't say: "Well, I'm now going into a weight-reduction program so when I watch television at night, instead of eating peanuts, I'm going to have a big bag of celery there." Replacing high-caloric foods with low-caloric foods is not bad per se. But the problem quite frequently is that you substitute a food you don't like. And you haven't questioned why you're eating at this particular time in this particular place; you haven't broken the pattern. Then, after a while, you're likely to say: "I really can't stand eating this celery." But you're still in the habit of eating at that hour of the day, in front of the television set, and you slip back to high-calorie snacks such as peanuts.

The food itself and the amounts are not what matter most, for they are only *the end result of all the things that lead you to eat*. To achieve permanent weight loss you must discover—and analyze—*what* produced the end result. You can accomplish this by keeping records. Indeed, you must learn to be your own observer. To keep records of everything you consume in a day, except for water, black coffee, or plain tea. To list the calories in each food you eat. To record the time you start and finish each meal or snack. And the precise place where you are eating. And with whom. And in what physical position—standing, sitting, lying down. You are to record what else you were doing while eating—reading, perhaps, or watching TV or cooking. And your mood; were you bored, depressed, happy? And, on a scale of 0 to 5, how hungry you were.

When you analyze them, the records can prove that you are an unthinking nibbler, say, or that you don't really eat because of tension, as you think you do. A pattern will emerge. Until one of our patients began keeping records, for example, she never realized she ate a little something, usually candy, every two hours. As a remedy we suggested she stretch the time between snacks little by little. "The first time I tried it I was almost hysterical," she said. "I was only able to wait twenty minutes. The second time I distracted myself by calling someone on the telephone." Eventually she broke the habit.

The records showed another woman that she ate a lot at home between 4:00 P.M. and 6:00 P.M. Now she leaves the house in the late afternoon to do her errands. Records showed a college student that, without thinking, she bought a pastry every day on her way to school. She realized she'd developed that habit simply because there was a bakery en route. She takes a new route now to avoid the bakery.

YOUR PERSONAL
RECORD-KEEPING PROGRAM

The first week you keep records, don't make any big changes in your eating behavior. The idea is for you to get a look, on paper, in black and white, of the habits you've been following for a long time. If you keep records honestly, you'll find out things you never before realized. And you'll no longer be able to fool yourself into thinking you've consumed less than you actually have. Self-monitoring develops the skills and attitudes that are the foundation of self-change, that enable you to break habits. It heightens your awareness of your own behavior, it increases the accuracy of your self-perceptions and, as a result, eliminates self-deception. If you can't be honest with yourself, you're likely to remain fat.

You may resist record keeping. It takes some time, and effort. But don't fool yourself by thinking you'll remember everything, that you don't have to write it down. You won't. And don't fool yourself either by saying the only reason you won't keep records is that you'd be too embarrassed if people saw you. You can always tell them you've got an allergy, and your doctor wants you to write down everything you eat so he can pinpoint it.

Suppose, when you start a weight-reduction program, you say, "I have fifty pounds to lose." And someone asks, "What does it take to lose fifty pounds? How much effort does it take to lose fifty pounds?" All you can reply, perhaps, is: "I don't know. But I'm going to do it."

Ask yourself now: "How much effort does it take to fill out a set of records for just one week? It's going to take me maybe fifteen minutes a day. It's going to mean that I'll have to carry the records in my pocket. Is that a reasonable thing for me to do for the next seven days?" And that's all we're going to think about—the next seven days.

Records Kept
at Our Clinic

At our clinic we supply patients with two types of record forms. The first is a daily food-intake record, which you see next.

FOOD-INTAKE RECORD

Time Start	Time End	Place	Phy Pos	Alone or With Whom	Assoc. Activity
6–11					
11–4					
4–9					
9–6					

Percent of entries filled out right before or after eating

Date:_____ Name:_____

M	H	Food and Amount	Calories

0   25   50   75   100

First we instruct all patients: Do not leave any column blank on the food-intake form. And then:

1. Record the time of beginning and the time of ending each meal or snack. An entry should be considered a separate meal or snack if there has been a lapse of fifteen minutes between bites.

2. Record the place where eaten. If at home, the room. If away from home, the name of the restaurant or store and whether at a counter, table, desk, etc.

3. Physical Position. Use the following code: standing (1), sitting (2), and lying down (3).

4. Alone or With Whom. If alone, write "alone." If with one or more people, write the number and relationship; for example, "3—husband, child, friend."

5. Associated Activity. Anything that you're doing while eating, such as reading, watching TV, talking, etc.

6. Mood. There are nine categories of mood that might occur just before you eat. Record your mood before you begin eating. Use the first letter of whichever word most nearly coincides with your mood: Neutral, Content, Tense, Depressed, Angry, Happy, Bored, Fatigued, Rushed.

7. Hunger. We want you to record your feeling of hunger just before eating. Please record any number between 0 and 5 that describes your degree of hunger. No hunger is represented by 0, while 5 represents extreme hunger.

8. Please record the name of the food and an estimate of either the weight of the food, the size of the portion, or the number of pieces. Next to the inventory of food consumed at that particular time, note if this was a meal (M) or snack (S).

9. Look up the number of calories in each portion and record them. We recommend the use of two pocket-size calorie books—one that lists brand-name foods and another that lists fresh foods. Or one book that lists both. Use the same books, or book, throughout the week.

When completed, a single day's food-intake record will look like the charts on pages 42 and 43.

At the end of each week we ask patients to review the seven daily food-intake forms and transfer information to the analysis form, which you can see on pages 44–47.

The analysis form is very important throughout treatment because it provides a summary or overview of a week's eating patterns. It provides essential information for planning individualized treatment techniques; it helps assess the effectiveness of these treatment techniques; and, for the future, shows patients how they can always analyze their own eating habits and the factors responsible for them.

The daily food records provide the information needed to fill out the weekly analysis form. Filling out the analysis form is not difficult, but it does require a certain amount of attention to detail. Some people like to fill out the analysis form at the end of

FOOD-INTAKE RECORD

Time Start	End	Place	Phy Pos	Alone or With Whom	Assoc. Activity
6–11					
7:10	7:45	Kitchen	2	Family	TV Talking
10:15	10:20	Kitchen	1	Alone	washing dishes
11–4					
12:52	1:15	Kitchen	2	Alone	TV
4–9					
4:15	4:45	Den	2	Alone	Sewing TV
5:00	5:16	Kitchen	1	Alone	cooking
9–6					
6:10	6:45	Kitchen	2	Son.	Talking
8:45	8:55	Dining Room	2	Family	Talking

Percent of entries filled out right before or after eating

Date:_____ Name:_____

M	H	Food and Amount	Calories
H	2	1 oz. Cornflakes	106
		½ Banana	50
		½ cup Skim milk	40
		1 cup coffee	
C	1	1 doughnut	95
		½ glass orange juice	50
H	4	1 slice pumpernickle bread	90
		¼ t margarine	25
		1 Swiss cheese	100
		Lettuce + tomato	25
		1 T diet salad dressing	25
		iced tea	6
		½ Bagel	80
H	3	Diet soda	3
R	4	1 oz. Swiss cheese	100
		2 T ice cream	50
		chicken wing	80
H	5	1 c Spaghetti	160
		1 c meat sauce	286
		watermelon	120
H	2	1 cup ice cream	250
		Total:	1741

0   25   (50)   75   100

BEHAVIORAL WEIGHT-CONTROL PROGRAM

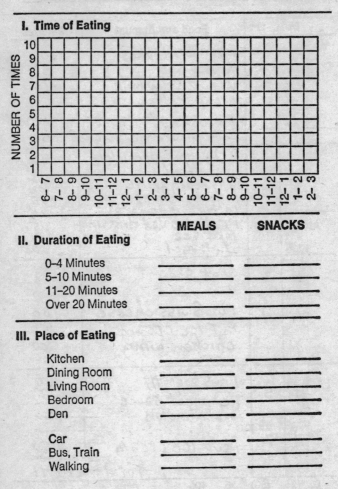

I. Time of Eating

	MEALS	SNACKS
II. Duration of Eating		
0–4 Minutes		
5–10 Minutes		
11–20 Minutes		
Over 20 Minutes		

III. Place of Eating

	MEALS	SNACKS
Kitchen		
Dining Room		
Living Room		
Bedroom		
Den		
Car		
Bus, Train		
Walking		

ANALYSIS OF FOOD INTAKE

	MEALS	SNACKS
Place of Eating (cont'd)		
Office	—————	—————
Restaurant	—————	—————
Friend's Home	—————	—————
Other	—————	—————

IV. Physical Position

	MEALS	SNACKS
Standing	—————	—————
Sitting	—————	—————
Lying Down	—————	—————

V. Alone or With Whom

	MEALS	SNACKS
Alone	—————	—————
Spouse	—————	—————
Family	—————	—————
Friends	—————	—————
Business Associates	—————	—————
Strangers	—————	—————
Other	—————	—————

VI. Associated Activity

	MEALS	SNACKS
Eating Only	—————	—————
Talking	—————	—————
Reading	—————	—————
Radio, Music	—————	—————
Television	—————	—————
Cooking	—————	—————
Other	—————	—————

VII. Mood	MEALS	SNACKS
Neutral	_____	_____
Content	_____	_____
Happy	_____	_____
Tense	_____	_____
Depressed	_____	_____
Angry	_____	_____
Bored	_____	_____
Fatigued	_____	_____
Rushed	_____	_____

VIII. Degree of Hunger

	MEALS	SNACKS
0–2 (None to Mild)	_____	_____
3–5 (Mild to Extreme)	_____	_____

IX. Type of Food

	MEALS	SNACKS
Alcohol	_____	_____
Baked Goods Cake, Cookies, Crackers, etc.	_____	_____
Candy	_____	_____
Cheese	_____	_____
Ice Cream, Sherbet	_____	_____
Jam	_____	_____
Jello	_____	_____
Nuts	_____	_____
Peanut Butter	_____	_____
Potato Chips, etc.	_____	_____
Pretzels	_____	_____
Sodas Diet	_____	_____
Regular	_____	_____
Sugar	_____	_____
Coffee-mate	_____	_____

Type of Food (cont'd)	MEALS	SNACKS
Bread, Rolls	_____	_____
Butter, Margarine	_____	_____
Cereal	_____	_____
Condiments	_____	_____
Eggs	_____	_____
Fish	_____	_____
Fruit	_____	_____
Juice	_____	_____
Mayonnaise	_____	_____
Meat	_____	_____
Milk		
Whole	_____	_____
Skim	_____	_____
Pasta Products	_____	_____
Pizza	_____	_____
Potatoes	_____	_____
Poultry	_____	_____
Salads	_____	_____
Salad Dressing	_____	_____
Soups	_____	_____
Syrups, Sauces	_____	_____
Vegetables	_____	_____
Waffles, Pancakes	_____	_____
Yogurt, Cottage Ch.	_____	_____

X. Total Caloric Intake

Friday_____ Saturday_____ Sunday_____

Mon._____ Tues._____ Wed._____ Thurs._____

XI. Techniques

1._____ 3._____

2._____ 4._____

the week, while others like to enter the data from the daily food records every day or every other day. Whatever the choice, the analysis form should include all the information from the entire week's worth of food records.

Most of the categories on the analysis form simply call for frequency counts. The easiest way to record these is to use tick marks to tally the total frequency. It is helpful to group the tick marks in units of five, with a diagonal being used to indicate the fifth entry (i.e., 𝐻𝐻 𝐼𝐼 = 7).

Category I (Time of Eating) requires a different method of counting. For each meal or snack it is necessary to darken a square corresponding to the time interval during which the meal or snack started. The time intervals are plotted along the bottom of the graph, starting at 6:00 a.m. The total squares darkened in a column will add up to the number of times during the week that a meal or snack occurred at that particular time interval. If a total of five meals or snacks were eaten, for example, between 7:00

I. Time of Eating

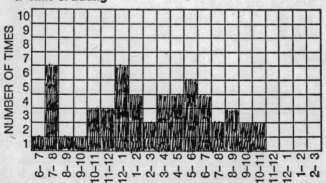

a.m. and 8:00 a.m., five squares would be darkened in the "7–8" column.

In the sample of Category I shown here we can see that one ingestion began sometime between 6:00 and 7:00 a.m., six between 7:00 and 8:00 a.m., etc.

This pictorial description is very helpful in that it provides, at a glance, both the frequency and the time pattern of all ingestions for the week.

In Category I there is no need to distinguish between meals and snacks. For the rest of the categories it is necessary to analyze meals and snacks separately. This is easily done, as can be seen in the following examples:

Category II (Duration of Eating) asks for a count of number of meals that lasted from 0 to 4 minutes, 5 to 10 minutes, etc. The same information is required for snacks.

We can easily see here that during the week this person had three meals that lasted from 0 to 4 minutes, eight that lasted from 5 to 10 minutes, two that lasted from 11 to 20 minutes, and three that lasted over 20 minutes. There were also twelve snacks lasting 0 to 4 minutes, six snacks lasting 5 to 10 minutes, two snacks lasting from 11 to 20 minutes, and one that lasted over 20 minutes.

	MEALS	**SNACKS**
II. Duration of Eating		
0–4 Minutes	///	卌 卌 //
5–10 Minutes	卌 ///	卌 /
11–20 Minutes	//	//
Over 20 Minutes	///	/

Category III (Place of Eating) concerns the place in which meals or snacks occur. Again, it is sufficient to use tick marks to tally the frequencies.

Here you can see seven meals eaten in the kitchen, two in the dining room, one in the car, one in the office, four in restaurants, and one at a friend's home. Five snacks were eaten in the kitchen, three in the den, one while walking, three at the office, and thirteen are listed as "other." "Other" is meant to include all places of eating not covered by the listings. Since the "other" in this example was a regular place of eating—the person's basement workshop—rather than a number of places, the word "basement" was worth noting on the analysis form.

Category IV (Physical Position) is a frequency count of the physical-position entries on the daily food records.

Category V (Alone or With Whom) asks for a fre-

III. Place of Eating	MEALS	SNACKS
Kitchen	7HH II	7HH
Dining Room	II	
Living Room		
Bedroom		
Den		III
Car	I	
Bus, Train		
Walking		I
Office	I	III
Restaurant	IIII	
Friend's Home	I	
Other *basement*		7HH 7HH III

quency count of the number of meals eaten alone, with spouse, etc. The same information is needed for snacks. Each meal or snack should be counted only once, no matter how many people were there. For example, a meal with spouse and children would be entered under "Family."

Category VI (Associated Activity) asks for a tally of the activities associated with meals and snacks.

Category VII (Mood) is a tally of the *dominant* mood, as listed on the daily food-intake records, associated with each meal or snack.

Category VIII (Degree of Hunger) asks for a frequency count of the degree of hunger during the week's eating.

Category IX (Type of Food) asks for a count of the number of meals or snacks that involved the foods we have listed.

For Category X (Total Caloric Intake) it is necessary to add up the total calories consumed each day.

And in Category XI (Techniques), list any special new techniques that may have been tried—with success—during the week.

CHAPTER
4

What Your
Food Diaries
Can Reveal

WHEN YOU ANALYZE YOUR RECORDS, ONE GOAL IS TO pinpoint those regularly recurring hours when there is a high likelihood of your eating. And in keeping and checking your records you also discover the periods when you don't seem to be drawn to eating. When you learn that there are certain times of day in which eating never occurs, you can ask yourself: "What am I doing during those hours that is obviously precluding eating? And can I do it more often?"

The time patterns of your eating can surprise you. One patient who ate consistently at six different time periods had always thought of herself as strictly a three-meal-a-day person, no snacks. But she was taking care of a bedridden, invalid father. And when she recorded her food intake, she became aware that she always nibbled while fixing and serving his meals. "I don't even like the food he eats," she said. "But I snitch at it, then later I eat my own meals, the food I *do* like."

We advised the woman to eat her own meals first. "That way," we said, "you'll be full enough not to be tempted by food you really don't care for." But this was a tough decision for her to enact. She felt she had to minister to her father before herself—and we weren't surprised. *We've always believed that if overweight persons paid as much attention to their own needs as to those of others, they might not be overweight.*

Pay particular attention now to your records of the amount of time spent at each meal or snack. Because, remember, if you eat slowly, you don't need as much food to produce a feeling of fullness. Also, consider the results of an experiment in which scientists fed several people the same meal, noted their eating speed, and an hour later offered them all ice cream. The ones who had eaten slowly were less hungry.

Savor your food. Be conscious of every bite. Make eating an event. If you are eating a meal in less than twenty minutes or a snack in less than ten, that's invariably too fast. We don't expect you to make a cracker last ten minutes. But it's not unrealistic to expect that six crackers, or ten potato chips, can. And you probably now eat that kind of snack in thirty seconds.

Even if you are having only an apple, put it on a plate. Core it. Section it. Savor it. One man we know who loves bread is able to sit with a single roll and take twenty minutes to eat it.

If you really wanted to ignore the experience of eating—which many fat people subconsciously do, because of guilt—what better way than to eat quickly while standing or on the move? To experience the food and the taste best you must not only eat slowly

but also eat while sitting down. Which is why we
want you to become aware, by keeping records, of
your physical position while eating.

We advised one woman to stop eating while at the
refrigerator. We pointed out that she was doing what
a lot of people with weight problems do, that she was
eating without paying attention to it, because of guilt.
So she stopped eating at the refrigerator. And gained
weight. Because instead of eating one or two things—
a couple of meatballs, maybe—while standing up, she
was now taking the whole bowl and sitting down
with it. That's not what we had in mind. Never eat
from a whole platter of anything. Put a portion on a
plate, sit down, and eat that. If you want more later,
get up, go back to the refrigerator, take another portion, and eat that. But make that extra eating a conscious decision, not an automatic reflex.

You must eliminate mindless eating. On the first
day she started keeping records, one of our patients
found herself in front of her picture window, waving
good-bye to her husband as he went off to his office.
She waved so enthusiastically she hit the window
with a bagel that was in her hand. She could not for
the life of her remember when she'd picked up the
bagel.

Have you ever stood at the refrigerator deciding
what to snack on and suddenly stuffed down a piece
of cheese to tide you over until you made the decision? Do you insist that the only time you stand and
eat at the same time is when you're tasting the food
you're cooking? Many of our patients do. Until the
records make them ask themselves: "If I'm cooking
spaghetti, why am I tasting the cream cheese, and the
ham, and the bread?"

If you want to sample your cooking, put a taste on
a plate, bring it to the table, and eat it. If you're

tempted by a pretzel when passing a street vendor, don't eat it while walking. Buy it, sit down with it, and eat it. Test yourself. If you really want a particular food, are you willing to take the time to enjoy it? Are you willing to take time out from whatever else you're doing to sit down and eat? If not, probably you don't want it that much.

You may be thinking, well, if I eat two or three snacks standing up, and they only add up to 300 calories a day, how important is that? Not very important—for one day. *But do that every day for a year, and it adds up to more than twenty-five pounds.*

If the records show you are eating in several places at home—the den, the living room, the bedroom—you're probably concentrating on other things while consuming the food. Pick out one place—the dining-room table, the kitchen table, some area devoted only to eating—and consume all your food there. This, too, will help eliminate mindless eating. And we find that if people stop mindless eating, this often cuts their calories almost in half.

Do not eat, then, while engaged in another activity. If you are talking or listening to music while eating, that's okay. All other activities may be distracting you, causing you to forget about savoring the food. Or you may be eating simply because of reflex, because every time you pick up the morning newspaper, say, or turn on the TV, you're in the habit of grabbing something to eat.

At night, after her family went to sleep, one patient would turn on the Johnny Carson show. And get an urge to snack while watching. "Why am I self-destructive?" she'd ask whenever she gave in. "I can do all right during the day when other people are around, but when I'm by myself, then I'm really self-destructive."

She wasn't self-destructive. She'd simply built up an associated habit: Johnny Carson had become a food cue for her. There's nothing wrong with eating. There's nothing wrong with watching Johnny Carson. It just did not serve her weight goals to combine them. She had to learn to separate the two acts.

Break associated habits. This will force you to decide continually if it's really worth having the food you think you want. If you have ten free minutes in the morning, are you going to read your newspaper? Or have breakfast? Or will you get up a little earlier so you can do both, separately? What if you want something to eat in the middle of the football game? Are you willing to spend ten minutes at the dining-room table?

HOW TO AVOID HABITS THAT TRAP YOU INTO EATING

In reviewing her records we found that one woman was eating in every room of her house, and always when cleaning. We asked her how she did it. She said she'd sewn special pockets into her apron so she could fill them with cookies, crackers, even soda. She had a little delicatessen in there. We suggested she get rid of the apron. And that simple act helped change her eating habits.

It is common for mothers to eat while feeding babies because they are in and out of the kitchen, near food. But they're not paying attention to their own food, so we advise them to eat at another time. Other parents automatically sit down and snack with the children after school. And often nibble while preparing the snack. We suggest the parent prepare the snack right after eating lunch, while not hungry, then leave it in the refrigerator where the kids can get it themselves. The important thing is not eating with the children after school but talking with them. The kids can have their snack alone. And then have a talk with the parent.

The presence of specific people may stir you to eat; that's one reason our records include the category called Alone or With Whom. And while you may not want to, or be able to, avoid these people, you may want to alter the activity, a card game, perhaps, or an evening's visit, during which you generally eat. "These records," one woman told us, "I look at them and, well, I never realized it, but everything I do with this one group of friends involves eating. We go to a movie, go to the theater, and we get together for a big dinner first. Then they always stop and buy food on the way there, and again on the way back. These people literally eat all the time. I value them, but I'm not going to eat with them anymore. I'll pick out activities for us that don't involve food. And that's the only time I'll see them."

You may eat because of the combined impact of companion and activity. Or companion and mood. Many of the things you'll learn about yourself from your records will come from splicing together the information from various categories. The psychiatrist Hilde Bruch was quite correct when, in a study of eating behavior, she quoted the naturalist John Muir: "When we try to pick out anything by itself, we usually find it hitched to everything else in the universe."

Record keeping must not be ignored during setbacks of mood or other crises. People sometimes dismiss a week by saying, in essence: "Gee, this was not a typical week for me at all. My son got sick, my dog got run over by a car, it rained for three days." We

insist there is no such thing as a typical week. We
want you to figure out, instead, what effect the sick
son or the rain had on your eating. January can be a
tough month sometimes, with rotten weather and a
lot of indoor gatherings conducive to eating. But the
problem is, it's going to be January next year too.

Because we've heard so much rationalizing, we
tend to grow skeptical. A woman recently said, "I had
a bad week," and we waited for the familiar rationale.
"My house is being renovated," she began, "and there
are three workers in there all day, and dust and dirt
all over the place. And my husband's sick father lives
with us, and the nurse just quit this week. And we
have a teen-age son, and, well, we just found mari-
juana plants in the basement. Then there's this rela-
tive from out of town. She went to the hospital for an
emergency operation, and her daughter came to live
with us." And our patient had gained several pounds
and was depressed about putting them on.

"Hold on now," one of us said. "What did you
expect? There were a whole bunch of things that
happened and understandably your priorities got
reversed; you couldn't put weight loss up as high as
you wanted. But I want you to go home now and instead of eating do something else you like to do—
maybe even, oh, take a warm bath."

"Oh, that reminds me," she said. "I can't take a
bath right now because the carpenters are working on
the bathroom. And I love to take baths. And, oh yes,
the macrame class that I enjoy so much hasn't met for
two weeks. And I love to sing and play the piano, but
there's so damn much noise and confusion from the
carpenters, I haven't played the piano all week."

When you feel overwhelmed, how can you possibly
deal effectively with your eating? If you're in a crisis
situation, of course that's top priority. But it doesn't

mean that controlling your eating has to suddenly drop to very, very low priority. Remember, in a crisis almost all people return to doing things that used to be comforting. Realize that you're likely to want to eat more. Work a little harder to anticipate eating situations, and to avoid them. But if you slip back, it doesn't mean that you've got no "will power," that you're never going to reach your overall weight goal. Don't let a few indulgences produce the kind of guilt that can lead to a hundred. And the records more than ever must serve as checkpoints.

The things to be learned from recording your levels of hunger are self-evident. The intelligence to be gathered from noting the foods you eat, the amounts, and the calories is pretty much what you'd expect, too. If you see, for example, that you're eating a huge portion of a high-calorie food—a big bowl of ice cream, say—don't think of eliminating it. But try asking if just one scoop less wouldn't still leave you satisfied—and go on, step by step, from there.

We find at our clinic that the successful patients are the ones who keep records, and are thereby quite aware of their eating. And the majority of patients are diligent. In looking over the records of one group awhile ago, we saw that two people that week had eaten a lot while lying down in the bedroom. We looked more carefully and saw that their times matched, and their foods. They weren't married to each other, and they'd been careful at the clinic to show no signs of a relationship. But on the records they were completely honest.

We liked that. But, of course, we couldn't help feeling concerned. We couldn't help feeling that what they were doing in bed was our business. Because in that bed these two patients of ours were consuming food.

CHAPTER
5

More Changes
to Make at Home

HOW CAN YOU AVOID EATING WHEN A SUDDEN URGE hits? What can you do to stop habitually snacking each afternoon at four? You can, in both instances, escape. Run. Get away.

The best defense against problematic eating is to change your susceptibility to food. You've already taken the first step by becoming aware of the forces that make you eat the way you do. But awareness alone is not enough. There are three other important steps. One is to change your exposure to food, another is to change the way you eat, the third is to plan ahead.

When we say, "Run, get away," we are talking about changing your exposure to food. That is, get it out of sight and reach. You can do this physically: Accept an invitation to lunch on your birthday, but not one to dinner too. Or perhaps psychologically: One patient was served a big portion of meat, cut it

60

in half, then told herself, "Half belongs to someone else and you don't steal other people's food."

It has been proven medically that the more we concentrate on pain, the more we feel it. The same with hunger, or what we may think is hunger. Don't sit in your living room thinking about the food you'd rather not let yourself eat. Do something else. Get your mind off it.

It's best to do things that get you entirely away from exposure to food. Don't run over to visit a friend who always keeps out big bowls of popcorn. Walk the dog instead. Try to avoid putting yourself in the position of having to resist food. The smell, the sight, a tiny taste will all heighten your urges to eat. Consider that, in sex, each stimulant—each kiss, each touch—increases the urge for complete satisfaction. It's tough—and awfully frustrating—to stop once you've started. Look upon eating the same way.

There are many ways to avoid food. For the person in the habit of eating while doing afternoon housework, we suggest a change in routine. Leave the house in the afternoon. Do the chores some other time. For someone who's up very early for school, comes home fatigued, and has a snack to perk up, we suggest a new means of coping. Take a nap. When your body is tired, what it requires most is rest.

If you're under tension, there's no need to relieve it with food. Take a walk. Talk to a friend. And when you come home from the job, wrought up, why go automatically to the refrigerator? Go to the den and read the mail. Relax on the couch. Shower. Get into a new pattern.

Do you eat when you're bored? Use activities as a substitute for food. Make up a list of chores you've been meaning to do—letter writing, gardening, bill paying. And undertake one when you're about to eat out of idleness. Make up a second list of things you particularly enjoy—painting, knitting, sewing, reading, jigsaw puzzles, whatever pleases you personally. Then stock up on the supplies for these activities, and use them, too, when you're bored or when you're about to eat in response to stress. But you must prepare the lists and supplies in advance. When upset, you may not be able to think of a project and are likely to revert to that older means of coping—eating.

Don't be afraid to refuse when asked to do certain volunteer work. It's fine for a thin person to sit home preparing cakes for a food bazaar, but there are other ways you can contribute. Similarly, work at reducing your exposure to food in your own kitchen. It's important that you begin developing entirely new kitchen habits.

First, we want you to get out of the kitchen whenever possible. You're probably unaware of how much unnecessary time you spend there, but in most homes a kitchen tends to be the command post. It usually has a table and chairs or a counter and stools where you can eat. There's a telephone and, next to it, the family message center. There's frequently a television set. And a radio. And a sewing machine. And a desk. And sometimes an entire family room built right alongside, with easy chairs and couches. There's a door to the outside that you generally use to and from the garage.

Why go into the kitchen to fill the can for watering the plants? Or to watch television? Or to pay the bills? Or to answer the phone? Or to let the dog in and out? No matter where you are, you may want to eat when you watch TV or when you finish paying the bills. But in the den, at least, you're not looking at a half-eaten chocolate cake on top of the refrigerator. The probability of your eating that cake is much higher in the kitchen.

The kitchen, ideally, should be a place for preparing food, period. It should not be the social center of the house, as it had to be in Colonial days, when it contained the main fireplace. It would be best not even to eat at the kitchen table, but to start using the dining room. You may be in the habit of saving the dining room for special occasions. We're saying that *each meal should be a special occasion.* Viewing meals that way will make you stop and think about food differently.

If you live in a small apartment, you won't have a dining room. But even someone who lives in one room can create some separation between an eating place and all other parts of the home. A little table can be moved around, perhaps, and regarded as a place to eat only when in a specific location.

Too many times people who prepare meals go into the kitchen at three in the afternoon and don't come out until eight. Ridiculous. Let your kids or spouse prepare their own snacks. If you're the cook and people must eat at different times, prepare all the food at once and let them reheat it and serve themselves. Get others to help you clean up. Don't pitch in yourself until you feel you're not likely to nibble. And if you simply love to cook as a means of relieving high emotion, at least be careful of what you make at those moments. Don't bake cookies, for example. Better to prepare, say, meat pies for the freezer—and to fix them so that they still have to be cooked an hour before they can be eaten.

HOW STORING FOOD CAN HELP
YOU LOSE WEIGHT

A patient reported she'd been in the habit of keeping a jar of cookies on a kitchen counter. While she was cleaning one day, she resolved to eliminate some clutter and moved the jar to the pantry. With that one move, made for entirely different reasons, she cut back her cookie consumption from three packages a week to only a few.

So, change your storage system. Make food less visible. If you absolutely adore the look of the cookie jar and want it on display, do what a friend of ours did: Fill it with dried noodles, which you can't just dip into and eat. Or, better yet, consider what another woman did. She filled her cookie jar with dog biscuits.

Decrease your exposure to food by rearranging your groceries. Don't leave food out where you can easily reach it. Store your food so that the lowest calorie foods are most accessible; the highest, least. This will not prevent you from reaching into the back of the refrigerator or cabinet. But it will make you think about what you're doing. You'll be putting some steps between the cue to eat and the actual eating. You should eat because you *want* this food, not because of a momentary impulse when you see it there. And if it's up on a very high shelf, you may have to bring over a chair, or step stool. Maybe you'll go through that effort six times out of the ten you get the impulse, where you would have eaten the same food the full ten times had it been out in the open.

Get pies off the top of the refrigerator. Get rolls and bread into the bread box. Don't keep crackers where you have to touch them every time you need the dog medicine. If you can, keep the kids' snacks in one cabinet and your spouse's in another. And don't rummage there for things that ought to be in your own.

Perhaps you ought to buy certain foods in small packages, even though the cost per ounce is higher. You will end up spending less money, actually, if you are the kind of person who, once the potato chips or cheese or peanuts are opened, feels compelled to eat until the container is empty. When you buy a smaller package, you have a built-in portion control; the likelihood of your opening a second small bag is less likely than that of your finishing an entire big bag.

Another way you can decrease your exposure is by repackaging the food you buy. Take a large box of cookies and rewrap them into small portions of, say, four each for storage. You can then say, "I'm going to have a package of cookies now." And after you eat those four cookies, you won't be able to automatically go on eating four more without even realizing you're doing it. You'll have to go through the effort of getting another bagful.

One of our patients very cleverly repackaged Hershey bars. She cut them up in tenths and stored them in individual aluminum-foil wrappers in a tin container high up in a cabinet. So instead of eating a whole Hershey bar, or struggling to cut down to a half, she was tempted—and satisfied—by only one tenth. She was particularly wise to wrap them in foil. When you prepare food for storage, especially high-calorie food, never use see-through wrapping. Always use something opaque, something your sight can't penetrate.

Use the same packaging techniques for leftovers. If you see them out on a plate when you go to the refrigerator for milk, you are more likely to eat them than if they're wrapped up. If you leave out a whole cake, you are going to slowly but surely, over a period of days, finish it off. But not if you slice it into sections, package the sections, and freeze them.

Think about what you want to do with leftovers. Are there enough to provide another meal? Or are there so few that all you're going to do is nibble on them? If there are enough for another meal, do you freeze them? Or can you tell yourself: "I've set these aside. These are for my meal, for tomorrow's lunch. I will not snack on them." Or if these are leftovers from a party, can you seal them up for use only at another party? If the food is identified in your mind as being reserved for a special purpose, perhaps you will not snack at it. But if you think you'll eat the food mindlessly, throw it out immediately. Don't worry about the impact of your waste on humanity. Make your contribution to world hunger, to poverty, in a more meaningful way.

Indeed, the same as you must learn not to habitually clean your plate, you must also teach yourself to throw out food. Better to dump spaghetti in the garbage disposal than to eat it cold at the refrigerator. Better to give away the peanuts your guests left—or throw them out—than to finish them yourself.

Take an inventory of the food in your house. Do you need all that? And if you say you do, are you possibly rationalizing? We've had people tell us they were stocked up on candy in September because they didn't want to be caught short at Halloween. And others say they keep certain foods around for the kids or because guests might drop in, but they ultimately admit these are foods they personally like. Do you bake or buy your favorite cookies for the kids? Maybe you ought to ask if there's some other kind they'd prefer. If you're really interested in servicing them, let them have what they want, not what you want.

Recently a patient who lived with her husband and one daughter took an inventory of her food supplies. She had, among other things, three pounds of cookies, two boxes of crackers, four half gallons of ice cream, a pound and a half of cheese, two pounds of cold cuts, five loaves of bread, two jars of jelly, various fruits, a large supply of meats, five quarts of milk, two quarts of skim milk, two jars of peanut butter, a pound of cottage cheese. *Cookies. Ice cream. Cold cuts.* Foods that are so easy to pick at.

"Why," we asked, "are you keeping these foods here?"

"Well," she said, "my husband doesn't have a weight problem and he likes the food. And I have to keep things for my eight-year-old to snack on."

Later she realized that just within the past eighteen months one of her children had left home for college, another had left to get married—and she was buying all this food out of habits developed when three kids were at home.

Reduce the amount of food you have in the house. And reduce the amount you bring to the table. Cut snacks into small pieces and bring them to the table in small quantities. At meals, dish out portions in the kitchen, and leave the serving platters there. If you want seconds, get up and walk to the platter; don't have it passed or brought to you. Just the physical distance of ten or fifteen feet can make a big difference in how much you eat.

In addition to changing your exposure, you must keep changing the way you eat, your table habits. So prolong a bit the time between when food appears in front of you and when you begin to eat. Our studies show you're likely to gobble food faster if you move right at it—and your aim, of course, is to eat as slowly as possible. If you're concerned that your food will get cold and unpalatable, keep half your portion on a hot tray. And plan a series of brief delays during your meal, just in case your stomach wants to signal you it's full. Remember, too, that if you eat slowly, it's tough for someone to force seconds on you. All you have to do is point to the food still on your plate.

Clear the table quickly after each course; don't allow dishes with food to pile up near you. Leave the table as soon as you feel full; let someone else go to the kitchen to scrape leftovers off the plates. We are occasionally asked: "Don't you think someone should have enough self-control not to eat the scraps left by other people?" We make no judgment. All we know is it's a problem for some people.

You are accustomed to saving the best for last, finishing the vegetables, for example, before the meat. Don't. Eat the best first. If you save the food you like best for last, you're going to make room for it. If you eat it first, you may leave over some of the other food, lowering your calorie intake at the meal.

Plan your eating in advance. Consider the day's activities and where food is likely to be. Write down what you will have. If, right before a meal or snack, another food appeals to you more, you might try telling yourself, "I don't have to have it today. I'll plan to have that tomorrow." If you do make a change, try to maintain the same approximate calorie count. And before you eat the new food, write the change on your menu sheet, even if it's only a few minutes in advance. When we say, "It's okay to eat when you want to eat," it's within this context. That is, plan how your chocolate or ice cream or pasta is going to fit in as part of your calorie requirements for the day.

Ideally, plan a day's food intake when you've got

time to check calorie figures. And time to think about your impending activities—and your menu. Do you want to have dessert with tomorrow's dinner? Or do you want to save dessert and have it as a snack later at night? You've had a craving for a chocolate bar. Will you plan to have it tomorrow, or the day after that? If you don't plan to eat it tomorrow, don't buy it tomorrow. Don't make the mistake of stocking the house with chocolate and telling yourself you won't eat any until Saturday. *It won't work.*

If you've planned to have a food, and you're sitting down to eat it, don't second-guess yourself. You've earned it. Enjoy it without guilt. And this philosophy can apply in restaurants and at parties and on vacations as well. As you will soon see, there are many changes you can make that will enable you to lose weight and still serve your needs for an active, satisfying life outside your house.

CHAPTER
6

Changes Away
from Home

ALL DAY LONG SHE'D BEEN LOOKING FORWARD TO DINNER. *Lamb chops, rare. Asparagus. Mushrooms. Chocolate brownie.* A tempting meal. One that she'd planned the night before and would prepare as soon as she arrived home. Nevertheless, leaving work, she suddenly had a craving. It had been months since she'd eaten a cheeseburger. Dearly, deeply, she wanted one now.

Instead of dinner, she decided, she would have a burger with bleu cheese. And as she walked, she began figuring calories. From her planning the night before she knew that two very lean lamb chops—five ounces on the bone before broiling—would be about 250 calories. Another 72 calories for six spears of fresh asparagus, 20 for a cup of mushrooms, 119 for a chocolate-nut brownie with icing, and 40 for a peach. A total of 501.

Stopping to check the calorie book in her purse, she noted that a quarter-pound of hamburger on a bun would be 420 calories, and a tablespoon of natural bleu cheese about 100. A fair enough trade—520 calories instead of 501.

She stepped into a diner and took charge. "I'll have one of your big cheeseburgers," she said. "With bleu cheese. And please don't put the cheese on with a knife. Use a tablespoon. Exactly one tablespoon of cheese." Then she looked around and said, "Wait a minute. Make that a burger with bleu cheese *and* bacon. And give me French fries. And a Coke."

She sat down, tasted the French fries, decided they were greasy and shoved them away. She finished her burger and Coke.

A few days later, when the woman told us this story, we said we'd rarely heard one that offered such a curious mix of appropriate and inappropriate action. When she'd realized she was going to give in to her craving, she'd done exactly the right thing—planned it as a substitute for dinner. She'd been quite correct, too, in figuring out the calories in advance. And she'd been assertive in demanding the bleu cheese be put on with a tablespoon.

But then, standing at the counter, she gave in to old impulses. She saw bacon on the menu board and asked for it. She automatically, because she'd been doing it for years, ordered French fries and a Coke to go along with her burger.

And yet, she was still able to do something that would have been impossible for her months earlier. She was able to decide, after a taste, that the French fries weren't worth eating, that she wouldn't consume all those calories without enjoying them. So she ended up with nearly 200 extra calories for the day—from a Coke and two strips of bacon—and with the hope that next time she'd be able to simply order what she planned, without even looking at a menu board or surrendering to old reflexes.

Plan ahead. That's the key to successful weight control. In restaurants. At work. On vacations. At parties. In shopping.

Shop from a list. Figure out exactly what you need for a particular period of time and don't overstock. Your eating habits, as you know, can be influenced by your storage habits, and your storage in turn reflects your shopping. So buy certain foods only when you need them for immediate use. You know which ones apply in your case. One patient of ours would buy cookie ingredients whenever she shopped, including nuts and chocolate chips and butterscotch chips. And when it was time to bake, she'd have to shop again, because she'd already eaten the ingredients. "From now on," she said one day, "whenever I want to bake cookies, that's when I'll go out and buy the ingredients." Of course.

Prepare your list when you're not hungry; you'll be more practical. Shop when you're not hungry; you'll be less vulnerable to impulse buying. And while your aim is to reduce your stock of high-calorie foods, don't completely eliminate it. And don't accept low-calorie substitutes if they don't satisfy you. Better to have one scoop of "regular" ice cream if it pleases you than two of "diet" ice cream if they don't.

Don't have any misconceptions, either, about foods that carry "low-calorie" labels. Although a food may be low in calories, it is not *free* of calories; do not gorge on it without checking the calorie count. Also check which brand of a particular food has the least calories. One company's eight-ounce can of beans, say, may be lower in calories than another's. There can be great differences. Especially in canned fruits and desserts. And different brands of skim milk can vary as much as 20 calories a glass.

There is no intent here to take all spontaneity out

of your life. If you're invited out to dinner at the last minute, you don't have to say, "No, I can't go. I've already planned my meal." But don't tell yourself, either: "Well, I'm going to a restaurant and my plan's shot. So I'll just wait till I get there and I'll look at the menu and see what I'm going to have." Rather, try to help pick the restaurant, or type of restaurant, and figure out in advance what you can have that will be compatible with your tastes and goals.

At the restaurant, order all your food at one time. And mean it. If you've decided not to have dessert, don't change your mind later. If you've asked the waiter not to serve a potato, and he does, make him take it away. If you're entitled to a full dinner but don't want the appetizer, don't eat it simply because it's on the bill. You can always, if you feel strongly enough, have it wrapped up to be eaten at home as part of a planned meal or as a planned snack.

When you have finished eating, give yourself some irrevocable signal. Put your napkin on your plate perhaps, and once you've done that, don't nibble at leftover food, even if the waiter is slow clearing the table. And don't be tempted by loaded breadbaskets or relish trays. If the corn relish is particularly good at this restaurant, put some on your plate and eat it. If it's not, why bother? When eating out, why use up calories by consuming things you can have every day or dishes that this restaurant prepares poorly? Instead, enjoy gourmet dishes and the house specialties.

LOSING WEIGHT ON THE JOB

Eating out with coworkers can create problems. You may feel you'll be missing an important part of the day if you decline, missing important trade talk as well as social experience. We suggest, then, that you try hard to influence the choice of restaurant. Most people simply say, "I don't care where we go. Wherever you want." If you care, why be quiet and get stuck at a pizza joint, say, or any other place with a limited menu? Suggest a restaurant where there's a variety, including low-calorie choices.

If you entertain people at meals and cocktails as part of your job, the best move, obviously, would be to conduct some of your business under other circumstances. You don't have to shift all meetings to your office, but if you could change even one or two a week, that would be useful. In order to avoid high-calorie expense-account meals but set up the warmth of entertaining, one executive we've heard of regularly invites clients in for early-morning coffee, served at a table in the office on good china (and just coffee—no Danish). As for those times you're out, eat at a restaurant you know. Know the menu in advance. Know the people who run it. Get waiters in the habit of putting the rolls next to your companion, bringing you small portions, anticipating special requests from you.

If you feel obligated to join your companion in a cocktail, be aware of calorie differences: White wine has less calories than Scotch. When ordering food, select dishes that must be eaten especially slowly, and leave a lot over. The other person would feel uncomfortable sitting with a sumptuous meal if you were on a fast, but not if you say, "This tasted great, but I'm just not terribly hungry today." Similarly, when it's time for dessert, don't say, "I'm not having dessert, but you go ahead." Rather: "I'm having coffee for dessert." Which may make your client less self-conscious about ordering cheesecake.

People eat while in the office too. Are you dipping

into the candy jar on that desk because you're in need of a break? If possible, walk around instead or go to the bathroom. A woman at the clinic reported to a new job and discovered that her new coworkers brought in food every day for communal snacking. "One of the things I've managed to do," she said, "is get myself a desk that's as far away from that food as any desk in the office."

The morning coffee break may be a valued social occasion. You can try having the coffee, but not the doughnut. If the doughnut is terribly important to you, ask yourself: "What can I eliminate from the rest of the day?" Perhaps you're accustomed to having an egg, two pieces of toast, and coffee for breakfast. Is the doughnut more important to you than all that toast? How difficult would it be to eliminate one and a half pieces of toast before you go to work? Make a deal with yourself.

WHAT TO DO ON VACATIONS

Business trips require thought in advance. So do vacations. Set reasonable goals and expectations. Perhaps you won't lose weight while you're away. Maybe you'll even gain a pound or two. But if you go on a two-week vacation expecting to lose weight and you gain during the first week, don't use that as a license to lose all restraint.

Understand that as part of long-term weight maintenance you will have to expect—and compensate for—the occasional gain during situations such as vacations. But by making preparations in advance, you will be able to exert control in any situation, and limit the gain.

A patient will sometimes come back from a trip and tell us, "It was a disaster. I gained a pound."

And we'll say, "But you went to this same place last year, didn't you?"

"Yeah."

"And how much weight did you gain last year?"

"Oh, seven pounds."

"So why is one pound a disaster? It's a six-pound saving in the same situation—and that's an enormous success."

A department-store buyer was going on her annual swing through the Southwest. In advance we had her fill out food records, reconstructing, as best she could, her eating on the previous year's trip. Upon spotting the problem areas, she was able to plan how to cope with them this year.

Whenever you're repeating a trip, try to profit from previous mistakes. And if you're traveling someplace new, try to anticipate. We knew a person who was going to France specifically to eat at the multistar restaurants. And we were able to help her plan what typical days would be like, what she might eat at these restaurants, how many calories she would probably consume. We figured out a way in which she would gain just a bit of weight on the trip.

Will you, too, be somewhere noted for gourmet restaurants? If so, and if you usually skip breakfast at home, why not skip it there too? Just because you're on a trip doesn't mean you must eat three meals a day. *Aim your eating toward that big fancy meal at night.*

Will you be at a resort where they feed you as much as you want? Pass up the second helpings. Don't linger in the dining room when you're through eating. Make special requests for foods that aren't on the menu but will suit your needs. And here, as on any vacation, keep your food records.

Are you going to a place such as Disney World or a state fair, where you will be assaulted by snack foods? Be sure to write down in advance what you expect to eat during the day. Don't buy haphazardly.

You can plan your day's food intake in advance anywhere. We recently advised one man who was going on a cruise that he was obviously going to be confronted with a tremendous array of food. "Look," we said, "the people on the ship know what they're going to serve way in advance. They make up the menu for the cruise before the ship even leaves the dock. So they surely know a day ahead of time what's going to be on that menu. Why don't you just go to the head-waiter and tell him that you're on a weight-control program and you have to know what's coming in advance, that you need tomorrow's menu today. We're sure he'll accommodate you. And then we want you to sit down and figure out what you're going to have tomorrow, and write it down. Otherwise you're going to go into that dining room and not be in control."

To take advantage of exceptional cuisine, learn how to bank calories. Skip a snack at midday so you can have that special cream sauce at night. Give up pastry in the morning so you can order *gnocchi* with your veal later on.

You can "bank" as a means of handling many eating situations. You may try to fool yourself by saying, "I'm going to be with my friends, we're going to be playing bridge, and everybody is going to be having a beer or a soda, and there are going to be nuts and crackers and cookies on the table, but I'm on a diet and I'm not going to eat those foods." Almost impossible. Because we're so accustomed to sharing food and using it as a social enhancer, we're bound to eat when everybody else does.

Be realistic. Tell yourself: "Look, I'm going over to Suzy's house to play bridge tonight, and whenever I've been at Suzy's house before, this is what she's served and this is where she's placed the dishes. And I know that under those circumstances I usually eat this, this, and this in these amounts. Okay. I like to eat when I'm at Suzy's house, so I'm going to skip a few calories earlier in the day. And I'll be able to eat something at Suzy's without surpassing my calorie goal for the day."

You can practice portion control too. And you can position food far away from you. And you can even say to Suzy: "Look, Suzy, you always serve regular soda. But that just isn't so good for me, so do you have any diet soda around?"

And Suzy may say, "No, I never keep it in the house. We can't stand it."

"Well, then, Suzy, will it be all right if I bring some in from my car? Because this is terribly important to me."

And it's unlikely Suzy will be in the least offended.

DON'T BE AFRAID OF PARTIES

You must come to parties with a game plan. One patient went to a party, ate more than 5,000 calories, and came away convinced that he'd lost all "will power." Not at all. He simply plunged into the food without thinking first.

If a good friend is giving the party, call in advance and ask what he or she is serving. Then you can very specifically schedule in the food you'll be eating. Or if you've been to a person's home before, you may be able to anticipate, generally, the type and amounts of food he or she will serve.

Figure out when you want to arrive. If the invitation is for cocktails at six, with dinner at eight, maybe you don't want to spend two full hours exposed to hors d'oeuvres and drinks. Arrive an hour late. When you get there, don't just start right in eating. Look over the array of food and decide what tempts you most. Try to find out what's going to be served later on. The worst thing that could happen would be to start eating food you really don't care about and then discover that they're serving your favorite dishes later. There is no way you're going to refuse those favorite foods, nor should you have to.

Hopefully, you've saved up a lot of calories for the party. You don't want to sit there saying, "I'm not going to; I'm not going to; I'm not going to." Because you *are* going to, and then you'll feel guilty. You want to be able to wake up the next morning and say, "I ate what I wanted, and I had a super time."

How, now, to spend your calories? Do you want to use a lot of them drinking? If so, then maybe you'll want only one or two hors d'oeuvres. Eat them slowly, really savor them. Do you want to pass up an alcoholic drink, but feel you'll be uncomfortable standing around while everyone else is holding a glass? You can hold one too—filled with diet soda or water or club soda with a twist of lemon.

If there's food in front of the sofa, position yourself somewhere else. If the hostess starts passing it to you, say, "Just leave it where it is, thanks. I'll help myself." There are tactful ways to avoid the food you don't want.

Which of the six hors d'oeuvres will you have? And

in what quantities? The best rule here, as in restaurants, is to eat the foods that are special. You can have chips and dip anywhere, any day. Pass them up now.

If you're at a buffet dinner, look over the food, choose what you want, and try to get someone else to actually fill your plate. Tell the person what you want, then move away from the display of food. When your plate is brought to you, eat it some distance from the serving table.

At a sit-down dinner party, follow the same procedures you use at home or in restaurants. And don't allow the hostess to intimidate you into second helpings. Simply say, "I really enjoyed it. It's delicious. I'm saving room now for whatever other good things you have."

There's no need to always accept large portions either. One of our patients was at the home of a friend who baked a cheesecake for dessert. He knew the friend well enough to be sure that if she cut the cheesecake, he'd get a bigger piece than he wanted. And he knew himself well enough to be sure that once it was on his plate, he'd eat it. So he said, "That's terrific. You made a cheesecake! You get the coffee, I'll cut the cheesecake." And cut a small piece for himself. It was a perfect way to take control of a problem situation.

Improvise. As he did. Indeed, the most critical goal of our program is to help you develop habits and solutions that best suit you as an individual. You cannot—must not—simply parrot our advice. One of our patients went to a party and ate her meal while sitting at the buffet table, next to all the serving platters. She ate seconds, and thirds, and when we asked why, she said, "Well, the only place to sit down was there—and you said I always have to be sitting down when I eat."

Come on now. Common sense. Exercise your mind and your personal options. That's what this weight-control program is all about.

PART 3

Activity

CHAPTER
7

Other Reasons
You Get Fat

MORE THAN 150 YEARS AGO THE FRENCH GOURMET Brillat-Savarin offered a correct solution to overweight. "Any cure for obesity," he observed, "must begin with the three following and absolute precepts: discretion in eating, moderation in sleeping, and exercise on foot and horseback." In other words, decrease food intake and increase physical activity.

Brillat-Savarin's solution still holds. And is as simple in its sum and complex in its parts as ever. To lose weight, as you now know, it is important to learn the factors influencing you to overeat. You must also understand multiple other reasons why you get fat—including the forces that may undermine your resolve to grow physically active.

It is not unusual these days for a businessman, say, to start his morning by using an electric toothbrush and electric razor and to then fix breakfast with an electric toaster and electric coffee maker. Next he goes to the garage, which adjoins his house, pushes a

button to open the door, and drives to work in a car equipped with power steering, automatic transmission, and automatic windows. If the skyscraper he works in has a basement parking lot, he pulls in there, gets on an elevator, goes to his office, and sits down at a desk containing a telephone, dictating equipment, an intercom system. He can literally be in touch with all the people in his corporation, and with the rest of the world, without moving from his desk. When he needs something, he summons his secretary, and she does the running for him; if he doesn't go out to a nice business lunch, the secretary even brings him a sandwich.

At the end of the afternoon he repeats the whole procedure: goes down on the elevator, sits in his car, gets home, opens the garage door by triggering the automatic electric eye. He has a cocktail in front of the television set, eats his meal, goes back to watching TV, then crawls into bed under an electric blanket, having first flipped the automatic switch to turn off the light in his front yard. Our businessman so far has had to expend almost no energy at all in conducting his daily life. Let us hope he is not now about to engage an automatic wife.

We have become servants of such technology partly because of biological biases. Our physiology, our biochemical makeup, was set half a million years ago, a short time back by the measure of evolution. It is likely prehistoric man faced unpredictable famine then, so he ate whenever he could and, for future survival, as much as he could. Like a hibernating animal, he stored all excess as fat, which is the lightest bodily tissue and the best insulator. Then he'd sit in his cave, stay as warm as possible, and use up his reserve energy—his fat—mostly in pursuit of more food. The

slower our ancestor moved, the more energy he conserved, and it benefited him to do so, just as it pays his modern relatives to drive automobiles slowly during gasoline shortages.

Our biological system would predispose us, thus, to eat whenever food is available—and to minimize energy expenditure whenever we can. Yet nowhere, ever, has food been more accessible and human energy in less demand than in modern America. Biologically, a person of normal weight can survive starvation approximately thirty days, and an overweight person, longer. But you hardly need stuff yourself today out of fear of that old natural-selection process, survival of the fattest.

As a species we share some basic biological predispositions, but there are great genetic differences among individuals. Although both eat the same amount, one baby may be fatter than another because, since birth, one has lain quietly and the other has constantly squirmed. No one knows what produces a sedentary baby, or a lithe, lively one. Nor does anyone know how to alter any of the genetic forces that may relegate somebody to a lifetime of fighting fat. But we do know that, despite them, *anyone can lose weight*.

CULTURAL FORCES YOU MUST FIGHT

Beyond biology, some of the same environmental agents that move people to overeat enact other influences on weight too. There is, for example, the effect of one's culture. In cultures where food is hard to come by, obesity has a positive connotation, signifying status, while in affluent societies, where there is an abundance of food, obesity is often viewed negatively.

Many immigrants who came here three quarters of a century ago were escaping lands struck by famine. And with food suddenly available and within their means, they felt not only compelled but also proud to fatten up. Back then, people came to regard fatness as a sign of health too. Because certain prevalent diseases, such as tuberculosis, turned victims consumptive, most scrawny people were regarded with some sympathy and suspicion. And the conception that fat babies and fat children are the healthiest unfortunately still persists.

In some cultures, as an annual tribute, potentates have collected their weight in precious stones. In ancient Hawaii kings and queens were force-fed, swelling them, by intent, to over four hundred pounds, as a sign of status. Body size became the most significant characteristic of these rulers, and perhaps the one likeliest to be emulated by a subject attempting to certify his own worth. Today you yourself may be fat because of the models in your life.

Various models have impact on you. It is our suspicion that weight, as well as fashion, can be influenced by celebrities, that Babe Ruth's success gave stout people an excuse not to reduce, that Winston Churchill's encourages "portliness" in England to this day. But people are most strongly influenced by family models. Children continually adopt the habits of their parents, if not instantly, then some time in the future. It is not inevitable, but it is likely, that a girl with a fat mother will be imitative by the time she starts raising her own family. And that a boy, upon becoming a father, will tend to act as his own did.

We have one patient, a man in his forties, who

remembers quite clearly a conversation he had at the age of five or six. "When you're a big boy," his father, a fat man, said, "you'll be able to eat a lot—like me." Psychologically that had considerable sway: *When I get to be big, that means I can eat a lot*. And indeed he now does.

On the surface this man's biggest problem is the quantity of food he eats each night at dinner. Before leaving work he will come home and tell his wife when he plans to arrive. The instant he gets home he expects dinner to be ready. His wife will then serve him, put the food back in the kitchen, and later he'll ask her to bring seconds. Seeing an obvious place for behavior change, we once said, "Okay, let your wife continue serving the first portion. But if you want seconds, go up and get them yourself. That'll make you think harder about the choice, make it less of an easy, automatic decision."

And he said, "Absolutely not!" He was loud and emotional. "When I come home," he said, "I'm going to sit down in my chair and I'm going to stay seated. I'm not going to go running around in the kitchen getting my own food."

It was clear that we were not talking merely of table habits. We were talking about the role of "the breadwinner," the posture of "the head of the family." We soon learned that his father not only had influenced the quantity of food our patient now ate, but had set a style of household command that was further contributing to fatness. Our patient had a lot to sort out in his own mind before he'd be able to make significant changes in his life-style. Most particularly, he would have to give careful consideration to what the role of a husband and father really ought to be.

HOW YOUR FAMILY CAN MAKE YOU FAT

There are more obvious influences family life can
have. If your entire family is physically active, you'll
have a model for behavior that will serve your weight
well all your life. You'll be well off, too, if your family
insists you do chores. But not if your mother waits on
you. And not if she regularly plops you in front of the
television set when you're very young instead of getting you to play outside. Kids can learn to be sedentary very early in life—and modern conveniences can
help them stay that way forever.

Once, when you were cold, you had to go out and
chop firewood and start the fire. Now you just go to a
wall and turn a little knob. Awhile ago when you had
dirty carpets, you hauled them outside and flailed
them with a rug beater. Now you skim them with a
machine. Until recently you had to trudge around
your lawn shoving a mower. These days you ride and
steer.

A century ago if you wanted to visit someone, you
walked a couple of miles. Or harnessed up your
buggy. Or rode on horseback. Not only did you expend calories in riding the horse, but also in saddling
him and feeding him. You had to carry water and
oats and hay. You didn't just cruise in on your horse
and say, "Fill it up."

Even the automobile required some work in its
early days. You had to crank up the car. And manipu-
late a clutch. And struggle with a stiff steering wheel.
And some days you found yourself pushing the car as
much as riding it. Now everything's automatic. Even
the decision to use the car. We had one patient, a college teacher, who habitually drove from one building

to another on campus. It simply never occurred to him that it was senseless not to walk three hundred yards.

In the past there was no electricity, no light bulb to extend daylight indefinitely. You went to bed when it got dark. You did not sit stagnant in front of the TV, eating. And in the past more people lived on farms, where you'd have lots of food but would work hard preparing it. If you wanted to have fresh chickens, say, for your meals, you had to take care of fences, haul feed, and learn how to slaughter. You didn't just run into your yard and pick up a freshly dressed chicken.

There was even a time when people climbed stairs. Now you use elevators—and in most new big buildings you can't even find the stairs, because they're designed to be out of sight and locked up for tight security. You'll stand in line at escalators, ignoring empty, adjacent stairs, to the point where now, at the new Philadelphia airport, they've built enormously wide escalators and narrow staircases. Most innovations in architecture, in fact, seem to indulge man's predisposition for inactivity. To save you steps on the streets, there are moving sidewalks. And someone figured out that in your home most dirty laundry accumulates on the second floor, where the bedrooms are. So to save you more steps, laundry rooms are being built upstairs.

In the face of this climate, under the duress of all this technology, you must, nevertheless, become more active. This is critical if, after a while, you are to continue losing weight.

Say you have lost thirty pounds and your body is now maintaining its weight on 1,300 calories a day—9,100 a week. To lose any more weight, you'd have to cut back still further. But remember, 3,500 calories equals one pound. How can you really deduct 3,500 calories over the week in order to lose a pound? That would leave you only about 800 a day.

The solution is to increase your physical activity. Eat 1,100 calories daily, but also burn up 300 a day through extra activity. You ought to lose your pound in a week.

The more active you are, the more you can lose. But so many forces are obviously inducing you to be inactive. Be aware of them. Be aware, particularly, that most technocratic improvements in your life are ostensibly made in behalf of efficiency—to save time. And ask yourself: "What the devil are we saving the time for? So we can sit down and watch TV? Or a spectator sport?" The people performing for us are rarely obese. It's the spectators who usually are.

Before you start any physical activity, though, we caution you again to check with your doctor, to get an examination and to ask him if there is any reason at all why you should not engage in exercise. And if he gives you the okay, start off by regarding the Yellow Pages as the symbol of all the opposition you are able to confront. You must never, but never—when your feet are available—let your fingers do the walking instead.

CHAPTER
8

Practical Ways to
Increase Activity

WHEN INCREASING ACTIVITY, THE SAME AS WHEN DE-
creasing eating, think of small steps, reasonable goals.
You've possibly not lifted a leg in sport for years. Don't
start now. Not yet. Consider, instead, some less strenuous movement. Every extra bit can be useful.

For example, some people wiggle around while sitting: cross and uncross their legs, shift in the seat,
talk with their hands. They use up about 25 more
calories per hour than people who sit stock still.
Wiggle in that chair only two hours a day, and you've
burned 50 extra calories. We admit that doesn't seem
like much. Except. In a year it all adds up to 18,250
calories. More than five pounds.

Of course, there are numerous other ways to lose
five pounds. Suppose you've been maintaining your
weight on 1,300 calories a day, a total of 18,200 over
two weeks. To lose five pounds, you can stop eating
completely for two weeks.

Psychologically and medically it is crucial to go at

activity gradually. Most often we don't even introduce it at the clinic until the seventh or eighth week of treatment; we realize that the mere idea of physical activity may be jolting, and we prefer you first focus on some other behavior change, something to give you a sense of success, a feeling that *ah, yes, I can control things*.

Don't start, then, by running around the block. And don't start any exercise at all if you've suffered shortness of breath, joint pain, cardiovascular difficulty. Or if you have chest pains, dizziness or faintness, gastrointestinal upsets, difficulty in breathing, any flulike symptoms. Or a history of high blood pressure, heavy smoking, high cholesterol, total lack of exercise in the past, or heart disease in your immediate family. Discuss any such situations with your doctor before going on.

The idea at the start, is to simply ease into an increase in your current activity. Can you walk one block comfortably? Try walking two. Do you climb a flight of stairs daily? How about doing it twice as often? We want you to regard activity as a pleasant experience. And if you make a sudden, dramatic change, you're liable to get unpleasant muscle aches and shortness of breath. We've had patients, for example, who have gotten all charged up, pulled out their old bicycles, and ridden away, only to discover their legs hurting so badly after a mile that it was impossible to get home. And they didn't want to be physically active anymore.

We don't expect you to switch from your new power lawn mower to your old hand mower. Or from power tools to hand tools. But we do want you to increase the frequency, duration, and intensity of what you are already doing. You can burn up additional calories by pushing the vacuum cleaner harder, by finishing the rug in ten vigorous minutes rather than twenty lackluster ones; your body, again, is like the automobile engine, consuming more fuel the faster you move. You can burn up more calories than usual by climbing to the second-floor bathroom even though there's a more convenient one downstairs. And by parking at the far end of the shopping center, as we suggested earlier, and walking the rest of the way.

Develop a new sensibility. Learn new options. Don't automatically approach decisions with a view of "either/or": *Either* I take the bus *or* I walk. Instead, say: "Okay, I have to take the bus. It's too long to walk. But I don't have to take the bus all the way."

Probably the best general rule to make is: Walk more. Walking slowly, at two miles per hour, uses up nearly 200 calories an hour; walking very briskly, five miles per hour, more than 650. By getting yourself in the habit of walking, you can produce substantial change in your weight. Listen, for evidence, to this man:

"I began walking to work because it allowed my wife to have the car. It was only one and a half miles, something like that. I liked to be outside anyway, and I was trying to lose weight and knew it would be good for me. So it became a habit. I did it in all kinds of weather. I never accepted rides, even though everybody would always stop and try to pick me up. It really bothered them to see me walking in bad weather; they don't want to pester me, but they didn't want to leave me stranded either. One guy finally said, 'When I see you walking out there, I'll blow the horn, and if you want me to stop, then wave and I'll stop. Otherwise, I'll just keep going.' That made him feel better.

"After some months of this we moved into the town. And instead of a twenty-five-minute walk, I now had only a five-minute walk to work. There was no way I was going to walk out into the country and back just for exercise. And I began to gain weight. Gradually. My first feeling was that it's inevitable, the old familiar story of losing weight for a while and then gaining it back. This confused me. Because I couldn't see any real change in my eating at all.

"Then I got hold of a table of calorie values for various physical activities. And I calculated, for the period we'd been in town, how many total calories I would have burned if I'd been making all those old trips on foot. My calculations showed a total of 34,510 calories. Or, 9.86 pounds.

"And I'd gained exactly ten pounds."

SNEAKING EXERCISE INTO YOUR LIFE

You may be intimidated by the idea of physical activity—and have already made excuses to avoid it. We're not surprised. At the clinic when we first talk about activity, people perceive it incorrectly: *My God, they're going to make us do calisthenics!* If you're out of shape, of course the idea of strenuous activity is frightening. If you've been fat since childhood, the thought of calisthenics brings on recollections of awful experiences in school gymnasiums. And even though you now know we're not talking about that kind of exercise, you may be summoning psychological resistance simply as an expression of your biological bias against activity.

So break through your rationalizing. Here, as with eating, be honest with yourself. We know of one woman who insisted she left the house each night for a one-hour walk. Upon observation it was clear that she did leave the house for an hour each night. But actually walked only ten minutes. And chatted with neighbors along the way for fifty.

Suppose you tell yourself you can't go for a walk because the weather's too cold or too rainy? Put on another sweater or long underwear or use an umbrella. Suppose you rationalize driving to the supermarket by insisting you can't get the food home without a car? Use a shopping cart. Suppose you say, "I can't go outside because I have a little child?" It *is* possible to bundle up little children and take them outside too.

Certainly, if it's unsafe to walk in your neighborhood at night, don't. But then you have to think, "Okay, I can't go out at night because it isn't safe. But what can I do right here, inside, to increase my physical activity?" Someone will say, "Gee, I can't walk up the stairs to my apartment because it's on the twenty-second floor." Right. But, once more, it's not "either/or." You can't walk up twenty-two floors. But you could get off at the twentieth floor and walk the rest of the way. We're not asking for a major behavior change, simply a one-inch change; move your hand down one inch—one button or two—when you start the elevator.

LOSING WEIGHT AT HOME
AND AT WORK

Think positively. Walking up a single flight of stairs won't make much difference in your weight. Not in one day. But hundreds of times add up to pounds. Even housework can take on a different significance. Do you regard housework as an absolutely horrible, tedious chore? View it now as an expenditure of calories. Every time you vacuum a rug or clean a closet or make a bed, you are losing weight.

Light housework uses up about 180 calories an hour.

Gardening burns 240.

Carpentry uses 230.

Driving expends 140; painting, 210; digging and shoveling, 500; sitting, between 70 and 100. If you stand instead of sit, you use up at least 10 more calories in an hour. If you are pacing instead of standing still, you expend almost 100 more. Every extra movement eats away at your fat.

We urge you, then, to become less efficient. *Less* efficient? Yes. Remember, extra movements burn extra calories. So if you do housework, don't save up chores. Don't stack laundry, but run it to the washer in small loads. If you're making beds on the second floor and think of something that has to be done at the freezer, go right downstairs to do it. Then climb upstairs again. When you climb stairs slowly, you melt 3 calories a minute, or 180 an hour. Do it very rapidly and you can knock off 10 in one minute, and 600 in sixty.

At work, if you're an executive, your secretary probably brings in the mail, cleans your "out" box, gets you coffee and sometimes lunch. Which is fine for her weight. Walk out to her each time you have a letter or memo for typing, don't save them up on your desk. Get your own coffee. And your own lunch. And don't always go to lunch on the most direct route; *you can eliminate more than two pounds in a year simply by taking a fifteen-minute walk each lunchtime.*

Move your telephone across the room; you'll have to get up and walk to answer it. Stand while talking on that phone or while working at your desk. Someone making a time-and-motion study certainly wouldn't approve, but how much, if at all, will these practices diminish your work? They certainly will contribute to your weight loss.

Examine your daily routine for other ways to add movement, and become *more* efficient in your very important goal of losing weight. Perhaps you can stop using the drive-in window at the bank. It takes more time to go inside and stand in line, but also eats up more calories. Possibly you don't have to buy as many stamps as you usually do at the post office. Instead, go there more often.

At a motel always ask for a room on the second floor. And don't park your car right under the door. Carry your own luggage too. In fact, get in the habit, everywhere, of using your own power. Use your feet instead of the car. The steps instead of the elevator. Question every labor-saving appliance you have. Do you really need, say, that electric can opener? Because *even the slight action of manually opening a can will knock off calories.*

Do things for yourself. Don't ask someone else to walk the dog. Make the kids do their own chores, but don't send them scurrying upstairs on errands for you. Make your own bed, if you don't do so already, and learn how to make it right: Walk from side to side. Get the sheet in place, walk around, tuck it in. Take the blanket, stretch that, walk back to the other side. Go back and forth for each pat, tuck, puff. You can lose about two pounds a year making one bed a day, fifty weeks a year. If you increase the number of steps three- or fourfold, you can lose more. And do a better job of bed making at the same time.

You must teach yourself not to worry about "status." Will the neighbors think you can no longer afford someone to mow your lawn? Or wash your car?

Or put up your screens? Who cares? You yourself will probably feel lots better.

A patient said to us recently: "You know, I had the most wonderful thing happen to me just in the last two weeks. I was at work and I was walking and I felt a spring in my step. It felt so good. It was almost a revelation to me to know that I could move like that." Yes. Yes, indeed.

How many extra calories would you have to expend if no one waited on you any more? An enormous amount. So, get your own newspaper. And walk to the mailbox for the letters each morning. Every step moves you closer to your weight goal.

Again, all movement can be meaningful. Even the act of preparing food can burn calories, but you'll use up many more if you cook from scratch rather than popping in a TV dinner. Not only will you be active longer—peeling, slicing, chopping—but you'll also dispose of still more calories while cleaning up.

Experiment with changes. Don't be embarrassed. If you sit in front of the television set three hours a night, you're probably watching at least ten minutes of advertising in every sixty minutes of viewing. Suppose, during the ads, you just got up and walked around the room. There's thirty minutes of walking. Thirty minutes. By just getting out of that chair every time a television commercial comes on.

CHAPTER
9

Fun
and Games

Dear Dr. Jordan:

I read in a recent issue of The New York Times *about the behavior-modification technique for controlling obesity that you and Dr. Leonard Levitz have developed.*

I would be most grateful if you could send me reprints of any journal articles you have published, or at least bibliographical citations of them. Though I am not a physician, I am an educated person and will be able to understand even fairly technical articles you have published.

I am the victim of intractable obesity. I eat as little as possible, generally no more than 1,500 calories per day, and exercise strenuously three hours a day, six days a week.

I am a tournament player in tennis, squash, ping-pong and volleyball and also play a lot of bas-

ketball. I jog and swim nearly every day at a local YMCA.

Upon receiving that letter from a man in the Southwest, we sent back a set of food-intake forms. We advised him to keep the records for a week, monitor his physical activity too, and send the results to us for analysis. He returned his completed records with another letter:

Dear Dr. Jordan:
Enclosed are the results of my week-long careful monitoring of my food-intake and activity levels. The results were absolutely astonishing. I found that I ate more—even in this week when I was consciously trying to diet—and exercised less than I had ever supposed. I found that I ate something like 2,844 calories per day, and even allowing for a 15 percent overestimate, I still ate more than 2,400 calories per day. Also I found to my amazement how very sedentary I really am. I am an accomplished athlete, and in the course of a year I play— play hard at, in fact—at least three sports: football, softball, baseball, swimming, jogging, volleyball, tennis, squash, ping-pong. Indeed, during the week in which I kept careful track of my activities, I played, for two or more hours each, baseball, volleyball, and ping-pong. But I realize, after looking over my activity schedule, that when I was not playing sports, I was extremely inactive, virtually always sitting down, either in my office or my car. I would have to admit that a moderately active housewife who doesn't play sports the way I do but does do housework, climb stairs, pick up children, run around the neighborhood on errands, and so on, ten hours a day, uses more energy than I do.

Also, now that I have taken a week to analyze my behavior carefully, I realize that even my energy expenditure in sports may be less than I originally thought. For though I am a good athlete, I have had to admit to myself over the last week that because it is hard for me to get around very well, I have developed idiosyncratic ways of playing sports to allow me to move around less than I normally would. In half-court basketball, for instance, which I played during the "monitored" week, I have to admit that I spend nearly all my time playing "pivot" and seldom move anywhere more than ten to twelve feet from the basket, while the other players run all over the court. Also in volleyball, which I play once a week, I cover less than my share of the court, and whichever players are positioned near me simply expect to cover some of my territory. To give a slightly different example, last night I danced for a few hours at a night spot here, yet I didn't do any fast dances, because I am embarrassed at how I look doing them, while many people did dance the fast dances. Thus, although I "went dancing" for a few hours, I actually expended far less energy than others who were there for the same amount of time.

This week of carefully monitoring my own activity, Dr. Jordan, has been a revelation to me.

Clearly, that man had grasped the core and the sweep of our work. And with unusual speed. Moreover, he had discovered what few people are ever able to discover on their own—that you can fool yourself about physical activity as well as about eating.

Not long ago members of a group at the clinic were figuring out ways to lose additional weight. One fellow said he hadn't used his swimming pool in years but was going to start now. And then at every meeting throughout the next month he gave us the same report: "Used my swimming pool three hours this week."

One week he invited some of the others to his pool. They went on a Saturday, had a wonderful time, and said so at the next meeting. But they also said something else. "You know how you use your swimming pool?" one woman told him. "You pour yourself a drink, jump in the pool, rest your elbow on the edge, and stand there talking and having a drink."

When engaged with honest effort, athletics can have multiple value in weight loss or weight maintenance. It can fill hours of the day in which you may have previously eaten or been tempted by food. It can certify your emerging new body shape, your new life-style. And it can melt away calories.

HOW CAN I BURN MORE CALORIES?

According to the studies made by a national food association, an hour of slow bicycling can burn up 300 calories, an hour of strenuous cycling 600.

Leisurely swimming uses 400 calories an hour, rapid swimming 800. Golf expends 250 calories an hour; singles tennis, 450, doubles tennis, 350; downhill skiing, 450.

An hour of slow rowing consumes 400 calories, fast rowing, 800; handball or squash, 550. Bowling burns 250 an hour; fishing and motorcycling, 150 each.

Karate will eliminate 600 calories in sixty minutes. So will fast dancing and jogging. And one of the highest hourly calorie burners, according to another source, *The Physical Fitness Encyclopedia,* is cross-country skiing (1,200). Remember, any of these vigorous activities requires good health and fitness.

Pick a sport you'll enjoy. Calisthenics can be terrific for burning up calories (9 a minute, more than 500 an hour). But for most of our patients calisthenics becomes a four-day phenomenon. The first day you do real well, and begin looking forward to a month's results. The second day you do the same. The third day something comes up and you either work out at a later time than you've planned or for a shorter time. The fourth day something else comes up, and it's impossible for you to get to the calisthenics—but you promise to do twice as many tomorrow. By the fifth day you've given up entirely, feel guilty, and are in the throes of one more "failure experience."

There are many reasons you may be hesitant to take up recreational activity. For example, you may feel self-conscious about your size, embarrassed to be seen in shorts or a bathing suit. At one meeting of a clinic group a woman said that her family was going on a skiing vacation, but that she herself did not ski, was not yet ready to learn, and would therefore get no exercise on the trip. "Isn't there anything else you can do while you're there?" someone said.

"Well," the woman said, "there's a swimming pool. But I'm embarrassed to be in a bathing suit in front of people. Most of the time I don't even pack it when we go away."

"At least pack it this time," another woman said. "Do that much for a start."

And someone else said, "I used to feel that way. But here's what I do. I have a big robe and I wear it to the pool, and just before I jump in, I take the robe off, and then I'm underwater and nobody can see me. And when I get out of the pool, I put the robe right back on."

After forcing yourself into such situations a few times some self-consciousness fades. Occasionally, a patient joins a belly-dancing class. Belly dancing is a fine way to lose weight, but a fat person needs courage to take it up. Most of the ones who do are reluctant at first, but they've established a schedule of priorities in their lives, and have learned how to be assertive enough to follow it.

Embarrassment at undressing for sports, or at engaging in sports, is part of a disheartening cycle. You are reluctant to participate in athletics because you're fat. And one of the reasons you're fat is because you don't participate in athletics. Indeed, the adolescents who need phys. ed. most are the ones who continually seek—and get—permission to skip school gym classes. These are the same youngsters who have unpleasant experiences playing among their peers; they are the slowest runners, the last ones picked in choose-up games. And as adults, they have difficulty even conceiving of themselves involved in sports.

Fat people who were slim and active when younger also may have trouble selecting a sport now because they were taught competitive sports in school that have little practical value to them today. It's awfully unrealistic to get up on a Saturday morning and say, "Hey, what a great day! I'll call up seventeen friends and we'll go down to the park and play baseball."

These days some school physical-education programs are emphasizing sports that can be useful later on—tennis, squash, golf, jogging, bicycle riding. These are the kinds of sports we recommend you take up. And we urge you not to necessarily reject a sport because you once had an unhappy encounter with it; you may discover an entirely different experience now that you're less overweight.

So wait until you have lost some weight before you

start in at athletics—and then go at it gradually. You don't want to run out in the hottest day of summer, say, and start playing singles with an expert tennis player. Take instruction first. And to help increase your pleasure and participation, try to get friends or family involved in your sport.

SECRETS OF SELF-MOTIVATION

Once, when asked to explain his success, the noted football coach Paul "Bear" Bryant attributed it to his players: "You can't make chicken salad without chicken." Of course not. And it's tough sledding without any snow—or sled. So if someone tells us she wants to start jumping rope, our first step is not to encourage her to jump over the rope, but to buy it—and this may take a few weeks because of inner resistance to exercise. If someone says, "Well, I could go down to the 'Y' and get in a volleyball class," we'll say, "Okay, that's a good idea. This week why don't you just call the 'Y' and find out the schedule and details." We were trying to encourage one woman to ride an old bicycle she had. Since we knew the bike had a flat tire, we did not start out by asking, "Why don't you ride your bicycle?" Rather: "When are you going to take that bicycle down to have that tire repaired?"

In changing your eating behavior you try to reduce the availability of food, try to make snacking more difficult. With physical activity take a reverse view. Work to increase the likelihood of your participating. Plan ahead. Be sure the bike is in condition so you can ride it when you get the urge. Be sure that the tennis racket and tennis balls are ready, that the court is reserved, that your partners are lined up. If you suddenly say, "Gee, it would be fun to play tennis," what are your chances of instantly finding people to play with or a place to play at? But you almost surely will play if the game has been scheduled a week in advance or, better, if you and others have reserved and paid for a court on a seasonal basis. Even if you don't quite feel up to it when the time comes, you won't want to back out if three other people are counting on you for the doubles match.

If you say, "I'm going to dance more often," maybe you will. But your chances increase appreciably if you say to your spouse: "Let's go dancing once or twice a month." And they are better still if you tell yourself, "I haven't danced in a long time, I want to learn the new steps," and then enroll in a weekly class.

Be realistic—and assertive. Don't say, "There's nothing I can do in the winter, it's too cold out for sports." Think of things to do indoors. During the summer one patient enlisted her son's friend to play tennis with her each morning at seven. In the winter she got her son to play Ping-Pong with her, and after the son left for college, she had her husband fill in. She didn't just wait around for her son or husband to ask if she wanted to play Ping-Pong.

Sports can serve a family well as an activity that brings the members together, and is good for the children to model. And sports can increase your eating options because, again, the more active you are, the less you have to cut down on your eating.

The effect of physical activity upon weight is clearly brought out by the problems of so many professional, college, or high school athletes. When they're burning up calories with two or three hours of strenuous daily activity, they remain in shape. But when their sport is not in season, or when they retire, they maintain their eating habits—and gain considerable weight.

If you want to eat more in a particular week, get more exercise. An hour of badminton will burn up 400 calories, approximately the equivalent of a glass of orange juice, two fried eggs, a slice of toast, and coffee with cream and sugar. Two hours of jogging will take care of 1,200, the same amount as in a meal of two loin pork chops, one portion of spaghetti, and, for dessert, a big dip of ice cream. *A whole pizza can put nearly half a pound on you. Two and a half hours of very hard roller skating can burn it away.*

Be careful, though, not to eat ravenously after exercise. Often, following strenuous physical activity, you have a need to replace fluid loss. Do not misinterpret this as a signal of hunger. Drink. Don't eat. And beware of high-calorie beverages. Would you rather drain a six-pack of beer now? Or be able to eat more at that great restaurant Saturday night? You must think about such things always.

Understand, too, the reactions your body may have after exercise. It may try to conserve energy by slowing your step, by producing an urge to recline, attempting all this not simply to restore vigor but also to cut caloric expenditure in compensation for those just burned. The body will fight hard to maintain what it has long regarded as status quo. And your obesity has long represented the status quo.

Probably you've not spent time thinking of this, but many overweight people don't keep gaining and gaining. Rather, there is one weight at which they stay most of the time and invariably return to between "diets." This weight has been programmed by biological and psychological factors, and when you start altering it through new eating and activity habits, you are going against familiar balance. Which is why you must be on guard constantly against the "old wishes" of your body. And why we next want to show you how you can correctly adjust to loss of weight—and how you can cope with all impulses to revert in the future.

PART 4

Adjustment

CHAPTER
10

Confronting
Your New Self

BY HER TENTH WEEK IN THE CLINIC THE WOMAN HAD lost twenty pounds. Nevertheless, she had a complaint. "Nobody noticed any change in me," she told us. "I wish somebody would notice."

We suggested a solution, and she followed it the next week. With the loss of only one additional pound, there was a very different look about her. We were not surprised when she said, "Somebody finally noticed."

"Well, you look different," one of us said. "Very different."

"Yes," she said. "I went out and I bought some new clothes."

It had been that simple.

For weeks the woman had been wearing clothes she'd owned when starting the program. Not only had their bulk hidden an emerging new shape, but their bagginess, their ill fit, had invested her with the look of a floppy old frog. She did not think it made sense, economically, to buy new clothes halfway through the program. But luckily she bought them anyway. Because without the reinforcement of people complimenting what she'd already accomplished, she might not have moved further. Because they provided her with new pride and ambition, the clothes absolutely had been worth the cost.

In other reducing programs you invariably wait until all excess weight is off before changing your wardrobe or your grooming. Not here. Our entire method, after all, is rooted in gradual life-style changes. Just as you must slowly make changes in your eating behavior and activity patterns, you must, too, gradually adjust to your new self. If you wait until the end, you'll be overwhelmed.

Recent studies we've made show that our patients do not feel the psychological upheaval that others do in so many weight-loss programs. The reason, we think, is partly because patients here aren't deprived of favorite foods, as in strict traditional dieting, but also because we move them along slowly, emphasizing adjustment in stages. The day you reach your ultimate weight goal should be no different for you than the day before. Weight maintenance should not require the abrupt development of new habits, but merely the continuance of those already formed.

A NEW YOU

By indulging in new hairstyles as you go along, by wearing new clothes, you are helping to certify your new image. You feel an increase in worth, renewed motivation. Your view of the work still ahead is not that of someone who, while studying, thinks: "Oh, whew, I've still got two hundred more pages to read."

But rather: "Hey, in just the last two hours I've already read one hundred pages."

New clothes can serve you in various psychological ways. As even these new clothes grow looser, for example, you're receiving a signal of further accomplishment; regard it as reward. If they grow tighter, obviously you must inspect your daily habits with renewed care. Yes, it can be a real economic strain to buy a whole new wardrobe every time you lose another ten pounds. But, again, common sense. Buy only a few things from time to time. Alter old garments. If you want to look your best, there are ways.

Throw away clothes as you replace them. Cut the extra material out of clothes when you alter them. Are you one of those people who go up and down in weight and therefore have complete wardrobes in different sizes? If you're a woman, do you have, say, a size-10 wardrobe, a size-12 and a size-14? If so, and you've worked down to size 12 now, get rid of the size 14's. And, later, the 12's. If you hold onto the larger sizes, it means you're expecting to fit into them some day, that your subconscious is saying, "I know this isn't going to work either." *If you hold onto your old clothes, it's a commitment to failure.* Throwing them away is symbolic of a commitment to stay thin. And if you do begin to gain weight again, prehaps the prospect of buying a whole new "fat" wardrobe will help you stop. Better that than seeing size 14's in the closet, easy to step into.

You can be driven by a fat psychological outlook or a new one. Often in clinic groups we'll confront those people who have histories of continual weight loss and weight again. And there will be dialogue something like this:

"The last time you lost weight, you couldn't handle it, right?"

Affirmative nod.

"Because you were still thinking of yourself as fat, right?"

Another nod, then an answer: "Yeah, I knew I was thin, people were telling me I was thin, but I didn't believe them. I still felt like I was fat."

Indeed, one twelfth-week patient reported that, without realizing it, she was in the habit of turning and walking sideways through tight places. She said that in one week alone at least half a dozen people said, "What the hell are you doing?" And it dawned on her that when she'd been fatter, she could only get through narrow spots by squeezing sideways. The practice, though no longer necessary, had persisted.

Similarly, a man recently said that "when I lost a lot of weight, I had periods that were really curious to me. I'd be walking along and see my reflection in a window or mirror and it was as if someone else was there momentarily. I mean, you see the person but the image you see doesn't conform to the image you feel for yourself. It was really amazing to me.

"I'd gone from a 42 waist to a 32," the man continued. "I'd go in and ask to try on some clothes, and the clerk would say, 'What size?' and I'd say, 'I don't know.' So he would measure me and then run back and come out with a pair of pants that looked like they were for a Barbie doll or something like that. It's really kind of a shocking thing, and I've seen it work the other way too. I mean, there's a person who's getting fat in middle age but really sees himself like he used to be and isn't really aware of how fat he's getting. And you see him in a store trying to pour himself into the same size pants he always used to wear."

We know fat business executives who are convinced their weight hurts them at the bargaining table. "I get in there," one of them once said, "and it's as if I'm actually thinking, 'I control all manner of things in my life, but I can't control my weight, and here I am, sitting across from a man who can, a thin man.' And I get the feeling that person is going to look down on me. I feel disadvantaged in the negotiations." This executive is one of the many fat people who believe that "as long as I'm overweight, I don't deserve anything, I'm not entitled to anything." When these people lose weight, they still have trouble telling themselves, "Here's what I want out of life." But unless they learn to do that, they'll continue viewing themselves as defective. And will be very vulnerable to putting back the weight they never *psychologically* lost.

It takes time and experience to learn how to change your thinking, particularly if you've been fat most of your life. And to best learn, you must start feeling and acting differently as early as possible in your weight-loss program. Right at the start we teach you to think like a "normal" person by showing you there are no "wrong" foods. We urge you just as strongly to change other attitudes and aspects of your life while you lose weight.

Not long ago, in a clinic group, a young woman said that her boyfriend kept asking her to go to his favorite discothèque, but she wouldn't because she'd been there once and, in her words, "Everybody else was a size six." What's more, she said, all those size 6's were looking at her and thinking, "What's she doing here with a fat pig like that? What's wrong with her? What's wrong with him?"

"Did you actually hear someone say anything like that?" she was asked.

No, she admitted, she hadn't. Just sensed it. But she did know for certain that people were staring hard at her when she came through the door.

"Now, wait a second," another woman said. "You just said, 'I go in there and everybody is looking at me.' Well, what do you do when somebody walks in the door? You look at them. I mean, you look at anybody who walks in the door. Why do you think you're singled out just because you're still a little fat? You're not singled out. That's just your perception of the situation."

"Listen," said one of the men in the group. "You really have to do what you want to do and not let the fact that you're fat or not fat influence you." He said that he himself enjoyed dancing, and when he was thinner, excelled at all the dances. These days, though, he only did the slow dances because he didn't want to feel conspicuous out on the floor. But now, he said, he was going to do whatever dances he wanted. He was going to be concerned with having fun, not with what people might think. And he advised the young woman to do the same.

Absolutely. If you wait until you're thin to do certain things—to get up courage to dance, say, or to go to the beach—you'll have just as much difficulty then as when you're partway to your weight goal; you're likely to be nervous the first time you try anything.

BREAKING DOWN OLD FEARS

Earlier you began practicing new eating and physical habits. Now you must start on new psychological habits. Convince yourself, for example, to go in and deal with personnel at a clothing store. And we suggest this for reasons that go beyond your physical and psychological need for garments that properly fit.

Many fat people have a great fear of shopping for clothes. And understandably. It can be traumatic to walk into a store, pretending your waist is 38, and have someone circle you with that tape measure and announce a 42. You feel ridiculed—and who likes to volunteer for that? As a result, many overweight people simply avoid shopping for clothes. The same as they sometimes avoid going to the doctor when sick because they know the doctor is going to point to the scale, whether or not they came for a weight check.

These are pretty much the same fat people who may go to a bakery because they want a couple of cookies and end up telling the clerk, "Let me have two dozen because I'm having a party for the kids. They're not for me." They explain too much. They don't feel it's acceptable to buy cookies for themselves, so they make up a story. But when you're buying a pair of pants, you can't very well say, "It's not really for me, it's for somebody else; I just want to see if it fits me." Ridiculous. You have to face the fact that you're buying it for yourself. And many people prefer to avoid the clothing store rather than face that fact.

But now that you've lost some weight, we advise you to shop for clothes as part of the process of learning to think differently. Even if you don't buy anything, go try things on. A lot of people do that day in and day out. But not fat people. A successful patient addressed herself to this in a letter to us, saying, "Ordinarily, I presume, one's self-image, preference as to clothing, hairstyle, grooming, personal style, develop gradually, through experimentation and absorption in oneself over a long period of time. But I never went through this process, first of all because there simply are so many things an overweight young woman, or one who thinks she's overweight, cannot do, clothing and hairstyles she cannot wear, limitations in the sense that she must buy what fits, not what she prefers. Self-absorption in a lovely woman can be charming or amusing; even when irritating it is acceptable. Vanity in a fat woman is ridiculous and intolerable.

"However, at this very late date, the program allowed me to go through this process of examination, self-absorption and analysis, and gradual molding of a more positive image. I have shopped, browsed, looked in mirrors, experimented with my physical self, and judged what is good and bad for my appearance more than ever before."

Many of our patients say with the greatest exhilaration: "For the first time in my life I was able to go into a place that sells only regular-size clothing and buy something." People who haven't had that experience cannot imagine the anxiety involved, the certainty that the salesclerk will say, "The large sizes are on the next floor," and then the incalculable delight and surprise of hearing, instead, the clerk's confirmation that indeed you belong here. "I don't think there's any way to describe the feeling if you've never felt it," a psychologist once said. "It's the same kind of shared-experience phenomenon that's found among people who nearly drowned and had to be rescued. As soon as you've described it to someone else who's had it, there's an instant feeling of rapport and understanding and recognition."

One woman lost fifty pounds in our program and, with another thirty still to go, decided to try shopping in a store that stocked regular sizes. She walked into one, said, "I'd like to buy a jersey," and the salesgirl said, "Yes, what kind of jersey?" This absolutely staggered our patient. In her old sizes, jerseys came in one style and in two, maybe three, colors. She simply was not prepared to choose among jerseys with various widths of ribbing, assorted lengths of sleeves, different shapes of collars, and in a multitude of colors. So she left the store.

Back home she said to herself, "Wow, I didn't know you could buy that many different kinds. I'm going to have to sit here awhile and figure out how I'll handle that." Obviously, this woman ought to have realized, simply from observing people she knew, that there were many styles of jerseys. But because she'd been too fat to benefit, she'd never before acknowledged, in her mind, their existence. She'd blocked out the fact, psychologically resisted it.

And now that she'd lost weight, there was a chance she'd be beset by a new kind of psychological resistance. A psychological resistance to her new body shape. Some people are very accustomed to using fatness as a defense, to regarding it as the reason they've not succeeded socially or professionally. And when they lose that defense, they feel uneasy.

Perhaps you yourself have occasionally thought or heard someone say, "Of course I didn't get the promotion. I'm too fat." Or: "Naturally I can't play tennis. What fat person can?" Or: "Certainly I never meet anyone at parties. Not as long as I'm fat." We all seek excuses for our failures. And blaming it on being overweight is so simple.

You may have grown accustomed to using your fatness as armor in other ways too. If someone asks for a favor, for your help in moving furniture, say, or in taking the Girl Scouts on a hike, you may be in the habit of saying, "Well, you know I can't do that. My weight." Now that you're thinner, you still may not want to help. But you must respond more directly or put more thought into diplomatic rebuff. And that's harder.

Faced with the loss of all those defenses, you're liable to be uncomfortable. That's natural. Don't panic. Realize that your discomfort can stir up desire within you to get fat again, and that here, as everywhere, if you understand what's happening, you're in a good position to master it.

We had one woman in the clinic who, after becoming thin, insisted on pressing for even greater weight loss. "I'm still too fat," she said. She was not fat. "I'm still too ugly," she said. She was actually quite attractive. But while her new goal was physically needless, it was psychologically understandable. For years the woman had convinced herself that if she only were thin, she'd have everything in life she wanted. And while one part of her was saying, "I want to get thin so I can have all these things," another part was saying, "If you do get thin, you're going to have to face up to an awful lot." So now, afraid to test her fantasies, she refused to admit she was thin.

Don't be intimidated, then, by grandiose expectations you may once have set for yourself. Now that you're losing weight, be more realistic, apply more common sense. Reaching for the ridiculous to make the point, we suggest you consider this: If you couldn't sing on tune when you were fat, why should you expect to when you're thin?

DON'T LET FANTASIES
MAKE YOU FAT AGAIN

Your fantasies generally are based on ends, not means. That is, you dream of the compliments you'll get when the new you starts to do something, but not about learning how to do it in the first place. You think about all the thin people you see excelling at athletics and somehow expect you'll be able to do that too once you're thin. Perhaps you will become an expert skier. You may very well accomplish that. But not without lessons. And when you take the first lessons and feel awkward, don't get depressed, but realize instead that everybody is awkward at first. Indeed, as you grow thinner, you must start taking steps to learn new skills and improve others—in sports, in interpersonal relationships, in all aspects of your life. You simply don't lose forty pounds and automatically become an all-around superstar. But if, as you go along, you have been making gradual improvements in various skills, you will emerge from this program not only with less weight but with new interests, new depth, new scope.

When good, inexpensive home hair dyes were first marketed, there was a rush to use them. What quicker, easier way to fashion a different look and, correspondingly, a new sense of oneself? Obviously, though, hair dyes produce no intellectual change, impart no sudden new physical or emotional skills. You can't expect all that from new body size either. What weight loss can do is give you a strong sense of accomplishment and impetus to move on to other improvement. And that is an important achievement—very important—in itself.

Understand, too, other misconceptions people may have about how life will turn around on new body appearance. Parties are not always fun. Being with popular people is not always fun. Reasonable enough. But the first time a person who has reduced is confronted by disappointment in such a situation, there's a tendency to think: "Damn. Was it worth losing all that weight for this?" That clearly is not a mature reaction, but it is a common one. And, in basic theme, a recurring one: "Why did I lose all this weight if everyone is not going to love me? I didn't have a boyfriend when I was fat; now I've lost all this weight and my new boyfriend only lasted three weeks." Well, maybe new boyfriends, on an average, last no more than three weeks—for everyone.

Any number of new social pressures may make you want to begin eating again, in defense. Don't be intimidated, simply be aware of the reasons. If you've been fat since childhood, for example, never had much of a social life, never developed courtship skills in adolescence, you may be overwhelmed by your sense now that, finally, you should become socially active. How? When? Where do I start? What do I do?

Fair enough. That's a lot of pressure coming from within. But realize it is possible to now shape skills you didn't develop in adolescence. You do not have a personality problem. Rather, you have some learning to do.

Go at it slowly. One patient who had lost a lot of weight felt she should be putting herself into situations where she could meet men. So first she went to a concert, which was a fine move, but the next week she went to a singles dance, which was not. By going to the dance she had put too much pressure on herself too soon. That is, there was a chance she might meet someone at the concert, but even if she didn't, she would still hear good music and come home thinking, "I had a nice time." But she could come home from the dance feeling fulfilled only if she'd had some pleasant contact with men. And she had not. And was devastated.

We advised that patient to advance her social experiences gradually. We taught her to be thoughtful about each step. To try to anticipate what might happen at each encounter and to be prepared for, not stunned by, various eventualities. And to be careful not to misinterpret reactions.

For example, if you want to call someone for a date and have had little experience, rehearse, ask yourself questions. What are the possible reactions to this call? If the person you ask out says, "Yes," that's clear acceptance. If the answer is, "No, I don't go out with anybody like *you*," that's clear rejection. But suppose the person tells you. "No, I have something to do that night. But thanks for calling." Is that a rejection or not? It can be, or it can't be. How do you find out? By trying again. A few more times.

If you keep getting refusals, there may be nothing there for you. But why? Try getting dates with some other people and see if you get no's from everybody. If you do, perhaps it's because of your manner, the way you're asking for the date. Get some help from a friend who is socially successful. Talk over techniques, methods of asking people out.

Rehearse. That's a good way of learning, and of alleviating anxiety. Many years ago one of us worked in a college counseling center where students sometimes came for help in developing social skills. In this one case, according to memory, a young man came in for counseling on how to call up a girl for a date. He just never had the experience and didn't know what to say. I had to go through steps of how he might invite a girl out. First I ruled out an attempt for a Saturday-night date. Too major a step for a first try. "How about inviting a girl in your class out for coffee immediately after class?" I suggested. That was easier, more natural. We rehearsed exactly how he was going to do that, and it worked out fine.

Next we moved to a Saturday-afternoon date. He liked to bicycle and he said he was going to ask someone out on a bicycle date. I thought he was at a point where he could go through the phone conversation himself. So we didn't rehearse. And he came in the next week and said, very depressed, "It was terrible. She turned me down bad."

I pressed for reasons, and it turned out that when this fellow thought of bicycling, he thought in terms of long, long trips. "Do you want to go out bicycling with me?" he said to the girl. "I'm going to bike to this town about thirty miles away on a day trip. Will you come with me?" She said, "What kind of nut are you?" But he wasn't a nut. He just didn't understand dating.

By talking all this through, by testing out ideas and by putting into practice a series of gradual steps, the young man became more socially sophisticated—and happily, proficient. And so can someone who, after long years of obesity, is ready for new social experience.

Social success may produce some anxieties too. There are people, for example, who have been fat most of their lives, now lose substantial amounts of weight, and suddenly are not wallflowers anymore. On the one hand, it's a tremendous boost in ego. On the other, they haven't yet developed a repertoire of behaviors to cope with this popularity. And they panic. And misinterpret motives.

A man may approach at a party with an offer to fetch a drink, and a woman may think, "Oh, God, he wants to take advantage of me." Such fears are sometimes reported by women at the clinic, and it is common for other members of the group to help convey some perspective. "He wanted to get you a drink? Isn't that nice? Isn't that flattering? Just because men flatter you doesn't mean anything else has to happen."

A lot of what we call "courtship behavior" is indeed serious courtship behavior. But there's "quasi-courtship behavior" too—a style of interacting in which people are slightly seductive, slightly flirtatious, but don't really mean it. Most of us can tell the difference, but there are fat people who have never had enough social experience to do so. "That man spoke to me. He's in love with me." Absurd, of course. But some people do have that reaction as adults—and we can hear the echoes of our own adolescence as we listen to them.

Here, again, it's a matter of building new experiences and skills gradually and not retreating, out of panic, to the familiar, to the old habits that kept you fat. Blended properly into your life, weight loss will serve you splendidly, will add to, not draw away from, whatever you currently treasure about yourself. A patient once said, "You know, in being overweight all my life I feel I've developed some personality qualities that have given my life a certain richness that perhaps someone who is thin just doesn't have." Because she was severely overweight, she explained, she always expected people to have a negative first impression of her, and so, to compensate, she worked hard to impress them with other qualities—her intellect, her humor. "Maybe if I get thin," she said now, "I'll lose those qualities."

No. No indeed. Nothing has to be lost. Except pounds of fat.

CHAPTER
11

Asserting Yourself
with Others

THERE'S A GREAT AMERICAN GAME, A POWER GAME, called "How can I get this person to go off that diet?" And some of the players bring to it an incredibly brute competitiveness. One patient, for instance, informed us of a woman who excelled: "This aunt of mine walked out on the diving board at her swimming pool yesterday. And tried to hand the person in the water a piece of cheesecake."

Thin people try to coax folks off diets. And fat people do too. Even a patient of ours admitted recently: "There's one thing I can't stand, and that is if I invite a friend to one of my dinner parties, why must she pick this Saturday night to be on a diet, the night I've gone to so much trouble to cook? I know that by Tuesday she's not going to be on the diet anymore, anyway, and it really burns me up.

"So I just don't stand for it," the patient went on. "I tell people like that, 'Now, listen, you go on a diet tomorrow. Not today.'"

The pressure from people trying to influence your eating may increase after you've lost a lot of weight. And other pressures may advance upon you then, too. Particularly, you may find your spouse, children, parents, or friends suddenly trying to disrupt the changes you've made in your life. But don't worry. It can be handled. And the first step is to understand the reason it is happening.

Equilibrium. That's the key word. People have grown accustomed to you and when you begin to act differently, it disturbs them. We had a patient who went out to dinner with two friends she hadn't seen in months. The patient had been very overweight, and her physical appearance had not yet noticeably changed. Nevertheless, halfway through the meal, one friend said, "There's something different about you. I don't know what it is." And the other friend said, "Yes, I feel the same thing." Our patient figured out what they meant. She was eating slowly, very deliberately, a new habit. And the friends were somehow bothered.

When you know a person a long time, you become accustomed to certain nonverbal behavior—the way that person walks, eats, moves, sits, expresses emotions facially. Those habits, and the person's appearance, blend into the fabric of your relationship. And when there is change, you may feel uncomfortable, because the equilibrium of the relationship has been disrupted.

Man, as a rule, feels most comfortable in neutral situations. Physically, you don't like to be exposed to sudden heat or cold. Psychologically, you don't like tension, anxiety, continual arousal. It's pleasant to experience temporary arousal; that's why you go on roller coasters. But part of the exhilaration is knowing you're coming back to a safe port, to the old comfortable level, the zero point. You don't want to ride a roller coaster forever.

People use many things to move them off the zero point, but they like to come back to its familiarity. And the same psychology can influence their attitude toward your weight loss. The feeling inside them, at first, is generally: "Gee, that's great. What a nice shape without all that weight. How exciting." But eventually it can change to: "When do we all come back to the zero point on this and to the comfort and the neutrality of the relationship that we had?"

It's less disruptive to, say, your marriage if you are returning now to a body size at which your spouse once knew you. But if you've been fat all your marriage, weight loss can cause disorder, even if in the past your mate continually exhorted you to reduce. Those exhortations were part of the relationship, even the battles, even such dialogue, perhaps, as, "How can you dare tell me how to control the kids? You can't even control your weight." Your spouse can't say that anymore. And there are unfamiliar gaps in your interaction.

BEWARE OF SABOTAGE BY LOVED ONES

Understand that some of the attempted sabotage of your new life springs from the urge, on the part of others, to bring things back to the zero point. Other problems can come from a partner's fear at possibly losing you now that you're more attractive. And still others from simple envy; perhaps the other person—a spouse, a friend—traditionally was the star, the center of attention, and now you are. The sabotage, no matter the cause, will generally come in two forms. First, through offers of food, inducements to eat. And also through psychological assault: "You've lost too much weight; when are you going to stop?" "You're not doing things the way you used to; I don't know how to deal with you now." And, even: "I liked you better when you were fat."

Gradual change, as we urge in all aspects of this program, enables others to more easily adapt to the new you. Nevertheless, there may be some attack and you must cope with it. You know how to lose weight. You know why you want to lose weight. Realize what your goals are, what your capabilities are, and assert yourself accordingly. Realize that another person can only influence you, not control you. You alone are in control.

Usually your self-regard will increase because of your success in getting thinner. And you will become by nature more assertive. "When I was real fat," a woman recently told us, "there were a couple of guys I was dating who would call me whenever it suited them. If I saw one of them one weekend and he didn't call again for six months, what could I say? I'd still go out with him. But now that I've lost weight, I expect better. I feel I'm worth more, and they can't treat me like that anymore. I'm nice about it when I tell them that, but it upsets them, anyway. Well, I can't help that."

Terrific. Too many people think it would be terrible not to be liked by everyone. But it's unrealistic to expect everybody to like you, and you must not always acquiesce to others out of a need for approval. In the great "get-you-off-your-diet" game, for example, you will often have to issue the message that, "no, I don't want to eat this particular food even though you worked and slaved all day to fix it."

One of our patients is a woman who's realized that, no matter how much she eats, she'll still be hungry.

Always. When someone says, "Come on, have some more, you're thin now, you eat like a bird, you must still be hungry," she'll say, "Yes, I'm hungry, but if I eat more, I'll still be hungry. Why should I be fat too?"

It is best to be diplomatic. In asserting yourself in regard to food, or to any of the pressures imposed by your new weight, be strong but not unnecessarily combative. Someone may say, "I made this dessert for you. I know that you like this. I know that you've been losing weight, but you're not fat anymore and you can eat this just this once." And you can reply, "Damn it, you have no right to tell me what to eat, I didn't plan to eat this and I'm not eating it now. I don't care if you've been working ten days on this." That's surely assertive. And hostile.

Suppose, instead, you say, "Well, that's very nice of you. But, you know, I really can't go off my weight-control program." Be careful. Probably, if you say, "I can't do it," the other person's reaction is this great old game is: "Let me see if I can make you do it. You say you're not going to eat it, then it's important for me, for my ego, to make you eat it. I'm going to keep badgering you until you eat it."

Now, what that person really needs is reinforcement for the ego, a lot of praise for the concern, for the interest in making something special for you. So it's best to say something like, "Oh, this is really good. Oh, just beautiful. Just look at it. Just wonderful. I really love this, but I just can't eat a bite right now. Can I take it with me?" And then you either plan it as part of another day's menu, or give it—or throw it—away.

In a continuing relationship don't expect that if you give in just this once, it will be regarded as a special circumstance. Quite the contrary. If you tell someone, no, you don't want anything, and that person keeps asking and you assent the sixth time, the formula is clear: To get you to eat something, that person decides, she must ask six times. And she'll do it again at the very next meal she serves you.

If you give in, you'll likely resent the other person. And yourself. Resentment just doesn't disappear. It accumulates, and after giving in enough times to someone, you're liable to begin avoiding that person, or you're liable to let out months of resentment in one angry confrontation. Don't wait for the big explosion. Learn to be assertive as events occur, or to deal with angers as they come up. Any kind of emotion is easier to handle in small measures.

PARENTS, PARTICULARLY, CAN CAUSE PROBLEMS

Parents are the ones who most often offer strongest disregard for your new habits. No matter how old you are, your parents' reflex is to treat you like the child you once were. And you, then, have a conflict: Are you going to act like a child and let the parents dictate, or like an adult and risk their disapproval?

We know a married couple currently living near both sets of parents. His parents and hers don't get along, and on holidays each set entertains separately and expects our friends for dinner. Through careful scheduling, these friends show up at each house, never admitting they've been to the other, and eat dinner both places. Which is fine, if you really want two Thanksgiving dinners. But not if you're rationing calories.

Surely, there must be ways to be sensibly assertive

in that situation. The same as there are ways to handle visits back home. People often will wonder why they go out of control when eating Christmas dinner at mother's. Because of tradition, we tell them, because of old responses that were set in childhood. Once they can realize that, they've made a start toward controlling the situation. Their next move is to decide that at a holiday dinner, as elsewhere, it makes sense to eat only those foods you really care about. Make room in your day's calorie allotment for those dishes that are special, but why bother with the others?

On a week-to-week basis, try to turn some invitations around. That is, even if you're single, try to meet with your parents at your house when possible instead of at theirs. You won't, then, have to cope with the pressure of turning down food from a mother who is standing, right in your sight, at that storied old hot stove. You'll also be in control of the menu if there's a meal involved. And while you'll probably have some problems with the packages of food she brings, that's better than problems with platters right in front of you, on the table.

Another solution is to invite your parents to a restaurant for a meal, to a place where you can order the kind of food you want. Or to insist, before visiting them, that certain foods be available for you. Or, if you're back home for a longer stay, to simply skip some meals by staying in bed very late mornings, perhaps, or by leaving the house.

As you grow thinner, as you develop new interests and discard some old ones, you may find your friendships changing. If your strongest link to someone was really that you were both fat and could commiserate with each other, that friend may try to get you to gain weight again. And when you resist, as you must, the friend may look elsewhere for someone willing to share misery. Fair enough. You can't ruin your life in behalf of that friendship.

You must be aware, too, of the potential dangers of certain other friendships. Just as an alcoholic can no longer hang around with friends who run to bars, you can't be with people who always focus on food. Either get them involved in other activities with you, or cut down your time with them. Don't let them lead you back to old problems.

Be prepared for old friends to be shaken by some of your new interests; if you swim at ten each morning now, the person who used to have coffee with you at that hour every day will surely complain that you're never home anymore. And it's natural for people to show some envy, too; when one woman lost weight, two of her old pals reacted by getting nose jobs. New friends, on the other hand, have no prior equilibrium anchoring the relationship. In fact, one woman lost sixty pounds, met a man at a party, went out with him four times, and on their fourth date he said, "I really like you. But you really should do something about your weight. You're about fifteen pounds too fat."

And she said, simply: "I am doing something about it."

A very diplomatic way of asserting herself

HOW TO HANDLE TENSE MOMENTS

The new horizons that come with weight loss are invigorating. Not only is there a feeling of accomplishment, there is a sense of potential. Invariably, our patients report delight with the expansion of their lives and with the new richness that can ultimately develop in the most meaningful of their old relationships. The conflicts with a spouse, the sabotage in an attempt for old equilibrium, are usually only temporary. If understood, if handled sensitively, the fears, the discomfort of those to whom you're closest can be quickly eased.

It is not uncommon for a wife who's lost weight to suddenly find her husband presenting her with a box of candy. For months now he's been in tune with her reducing needs, but abruptly he's come home with candy or cake or cashews. "Look," he's invariably told, "you know we shouldn't have this in the house." And he'll say, "Well, this was a special occasion." Or: "I really wanted some of this myself." Or: "We've got guests coming." And mean it.

Except. Down inside, his motive is to restore equilibrium. Be careful if a spouse suddenly starts bringing sweets home or begins preparing dishes not on your planned menu. Be careful if children start demanding that certain foods be stocked in the house again or surprise you by, say, cooking lasagna on a night you'd planned a light salad for dinner. They may have likely been driven, in each of these situations, not by a physical need for old foods, but by a psychological need for the old, fat you.

Possibly you'll succumb in those situations. Probably you love those sweets or that lasagna—and anyway, how do you coldly turn down food your child has cooked? If you give in, okay, but head off repetition. Take the child aside and explain, gently, that, "I really love it when you prepare something to surprise me with. Maybe we can decide the kinds of foods that you could surprise me with in the future, foods that would help me to continue to lose weight."

You must confront your spouse in an equally sensitive manner. Wait for an appropriate time. Never do

it when there's tension in the family or aroused emotions; you'll only escalate the friction. Wait for a calm
moment, when you're both content and relaxed. Then
talk.

And, remember, preparation can reduce tension. If
you rehearse what's likely to happen, you will be better able to cope when you encounter it. Let's suppose
a woman has decided not to have cookies in the house
anymore. She's made the decision without telling anyone, but she knows that one of these days her husband will want a cookie, and will complain. Right
now, she can sit down and rehearse, tell herself,
"Look, I know that once a week he asks for a cookie.
And I know it's not going to be there the next time he
asks for it. So what do I think is going to happen?" If
the answer is, "Probably he'll explode," she must
prepare to face it and think of ways to minimize it.
She should rehearse what she'll say. Perhaps: "Dear,
I've lost twenty pounds. One of the reasons I was so
fat was that I always consumed a great number of
calories simply by eating away at the supply of cookies I kept around. I've found that if cookies aren't in
the house, I don't miss them. I don't even want one if
they're not here. I understand that occasionally you
would like to have a cookie. My problem is that when
they're in the house, I would like them five times a
day. So I balanced all that. And I decided that the
best thing for both of us was not to have cookies in
the house. Not because I wanted to deprive you of
the cookie, but because I think you like me better
when I'm not fat. And I like myself better."

How upset can anyone get at such a rational, loving
explanation?

Recently a patient told us, "When my husband was
away on a trip last week and I was cooking only for
myself, I suddenly realized that my eating behavior

in his absence was the kind I used to have when I was single and thin." And she burst into tears. She had discovered that for twenty years she had been subjugating herself. And she didn't know how to bring it up with her husband. "There's no way I can tell him," she insisted. We said, "Do you think if you sat down and explained to him that you've learned this in a scientific study of human behavior, it would be okay?" She finally said, "Yes." And then came back and told us, "My God, he told me that of course it was okay to eat whatever I want for dinner."

Another patient, who'd enrolled in a heavy schedule of college night classes, found that if he had an early dinner, he was able to skip snacking in the evening completely. The classes occupied him from early evening to late, and once he arrived home, he was able to go to bed without wanting food. Unless his wife was eating, or had left out food from her snacks. Then he was tempted, and usually gave in.

His solution was perfect. He asked her, "Please, if you're going to eat at night, will you do it while I'm in school? And put all the food away, clean up the leftovers, before I get home?"

It was a reasonable request, and a reasonable woman had to honor it.

If you're unreasonable, if you say, "I don't care what the hell you think, this is the way I'm going to do things," you're likely to be responded to in kind. Because the nerves of your mate are more jangled than yours these days. You're the one who suddenly has become more physically attractive. And your spouse likely finds this threatening.

It can be very comfortable to be married to someone who is overweight and not sought after sexually. And when that person loses weight, it can be jarring. A husband suddenly has the feeling, say, that, "Wow, she's much more attractive to my friends, colleagues, and total strangers." Previously, at parties, men didn't pay much attention to his wife. Now she's better groomed, wearing nice-fitting clothes, and thinner. And he sees friends of his who've always ignored his wife, talking with her in the corner, dancing with her, laughing with her. This can be very upsetting. "Wait a minute. This is a threat to me now. Maybe I'll lose her."

You must realize that any spouse may have such feelings, no matter how good the marriage. And you must make a particular effort to assert your love, to display affection, to offer reassurance that walking out is the last thing on your mind.

Do not, by any means, pick this time to criticize. One man who had lost considerable weight at the clinic was getting ready to go out to a party with his wife. She was a fat woman, who hadn't tried to lose weight when he did, and now, as she stepped toward the door, he said, "I don't think that coat looks good on you."

Her thought instantly was: "You don't like the way I look. You think I'm too fat. You're such a smart-ass now that you've lost weight and I haven't." And right there, at the front door, it was World War III.

What a time to criticize her. When she's on her way to a party and probably feels that, in contrast to her rejuvenated husband, she really looks frumpy. People generally perceive the thin person as being "courtship ready," and the fat one as not being interested. And so here is this woman, perhaps feeling inside: "He's getting ready to pull out. He's getting ready for courtship again and I'm not." And instead of reassuring her that he wasn't thinking that at all, instead of letting her know how important she was to him, the man criticizes the way she looks.

Clearly, he should have been sensitive enough to have imagined himself in her position. Can you imagine your own feelings if your mate suddenly became physically attractive and began criticizing your appearance? The first thing you'd likely want to do, and quite naturally, is get that person fat again. Fast.

CHAPTER
12

Coping with
the Future

YEARS AGO, WATCHING THE OLD MELODRAMAS, IT WAS
easy to pick out the villain. Not only would he be
wearing black and twirling a waxed moustache, but he
had another recurring characteristic: his body size.
The villain, traditionally, was thin.

Years ago, too, according to a friend of ours, "My
grandfather had one rule he always followed in
business." That rule was: "Never deal with a thin
banker."

Villains now come in an assortment of shapes. And
sensibilities have changed since the time when corpu-
lence personified prosperity and stability. The successful banker these days is, in image anyway, gray at
the temples and flat at the stomach. Thin people seem
to get the promotions at work more easily than fat
ones do. The joys of losing weight—particularly if
your life-style changes too—can be far-reaching. "Oh,
yes, I forgot to tell you," a former patient said at the
end of a one-year follow-up interview. "Since I fin-

ished the program, I quit smoking too. And I got off the pills that I'd been on fifteen years." Indeed, our patients invariably enjoy life more after weight loss, are more content. Better thinner than fat.

But you don't have to be convinced of that, do you? Because your tendency—if you are like most of our patients—is to not only want to lose weight, but to never want to stop losing. And, emphatically, there is a time when you must stop.

Why the need to continue after reaching a reasonable goal? Primarily because in this society there's an attitude that "change signifies success, standing still does not." Each week, for months now, you've had the reward of seeing the scale drop. How exhilarating, especially if all your life you've wanted to see that needle moving downward. You just can't get that same feeling of accomplishment, that reinforcement, from seeing the scale stay the same week after week.

For a while there's compensation in the compliments you get. It is reinforcing to hear how different you look, how good. But eventually your old friends and acquaintances will stop commenting on your new shape. And you may find yourself thinking, "Hey, probably I ought to lose another pound or two," simply out of a need for some visible reward.

Strive for a weight where you feel comfortable. Don't impose more loss on yourself simply for reward. Don't starve off an extra few pounds because you suddenly see some chart with a list of "ideal body weights." Don't push for another five pounds because your body image is not precisely what you dreamed it would be, not if it means intolerable sacrifice to lose those pounds; weight loss alone won't redistribute all the contours of your body.

Be reasonable. Suppose you've set 130 pounds as your goal, and you're at 135 and finding it torturous to hit a balance of calorie intake and activity that will enable you to lose more. Stop for a while. Live at 135 and see if you can't be happy at that weight. If it's simply a matter of five pounds, you may be the only one perceiving yourself as fat anyway. No need to strive to be a stick.

Perhaps you'll decide that it's manageable for you to be at 130 during the summer, when you're more physically active. And at 135 other times of the year. Fair enough. Don't be neurotic about hitting a goal simply because you set it months ago.

THE KEY TO KEEPING WEIGHT OFF

What you're striving for is a weight you can maintain permanently through a certain diligence but not through torture. And the key to weight maintenance is to keep following the basic life-style you've established while losing weight. Remember, the day after you reach your ultimate weight goal should not be appreciably different from the day before.

Day-to-day record keeping will not be a regular part of your weight-maintenance program. Rather, you will have "internalized" the process; will be able to reflexively hit the right calorie-activity balance; be able to plan in your mind the foods you can eat in a day; be able to instinctively know where to go, what to avoid; will have mastered the knack of eating slowly and other important habits. It makes sense, then, to try to lose your last few pounds without keeping records. If you use the scale as a checkpoint, trial and error ought to eventually produce the correct "internalized" record keeping necessary for the last surge of weight loss and, then, for weight maintenance. Of course, if you see sharp gain the week after you stop keeping the records, start up again, go back, at the least, to keeping written records of your calories.

Some patients prefer never to stop writing down their calories. That is exclusively an individual decision. There is, however, one rule we consider mandatory: You must never forget that you've had a weight problem, that you have to be more careful at 125 pounds, say, than the person who's been 125 an entire lifetime. You must compute a calorie-activity balance that will enable you to maintain those 125 pounds and must foresee continuing that method of maintenance the rest of your life.

In all other regards consider yourself similar to any 125-pounder, and don't be self-conscious about your past. There are some people who feel compelled to explain every action: "I'm Sally and I used to have a weight problem." Nonsense. And if the subject of weight does come up, there's no need for full confessional. The reaction to you, if you persist in publicly looking back, is likely to be negative. In essence: "This person thinks he has so much will power, so much self-control." Or, perhaps: "Wow, what a fanatic. Just like my uncle about his operation. What a bore." And possibly: "Look at this hopeless case who's got her weight problem just barely under control."

Enjoy a fuller life—the freedom of movement, the many choices of dress and activity, the invigoration of fresh opportunity. By savoring the new possibilities in your life you'll no longer be judging your worth largely by the measure of the chocolate cake you did or did not eat. You will be valuing, instead, the hobbies you may have lately taken up, or perhaps the part-time return to school, or your new social life or career. More and more, in other words, the changes you began making while losing weight will form the core of your life.

One patient, a man who came to us after a heart attack, lost a lot of weight and, in the process, decided he no longer felt like dealing with the long hours and pressures of his job. "I'm only going to work four days a week," he told his business partners. "And only on certain accounts. If that's not acceptable, I'll understand, but I'll have to quit." The loss of weight itself hadn't prompted his decision, nor had the heart attack by itself, nor necessarily had the combination of the two; if, in response to the heart attack, he'd lost forty pounds on a traditional diet, he might still be on his old job. But here, the very first thing he heard was: "Okay, you have a weight problem. We now have to consider your life as a whole." And in inspecting his life, he'd discovered new perspective.

HOW TO ANTICIPATE TROUBLE

Periodically during weight maintenance—once a year, say—you ought to get a physical examination and let the doctor know about your maintenance program. Periodically too—perhaps for one week a year—you ought to return to record keeping. You spent a lot of time creating order in your eating habits when you began losing weight, but some disorder may have evolved since then, and record keeping will make you aware of it; you may, for example, not be eating enough extra calories to produce weight gain, but you may occasionally be eating while walking down the street, slipping back into a bad old habit. Think in terms of a garden upon which you expend a lot of energy early in the season but later ignore. The weeds may not do harm right away, but they will after a while.

Weigh yourself each week. And determine in advance how much successive weight gain ought to command your concern and action. Don't ever say, "Well, it's only been two pounds this week," and then, a month later, "Well, that's only two more pounds." That's how weight insidiously comes back. You must have a cutoff point at which you say, "Wait a minute. I must be slipping somewhere. Now I have to look back and see where the habits are falling apart. Is my activity level down because it's a particular time of year? Have I just gone through a holiday? Am I starting to eat in situations where for a long period of time I hadn't?" To precisely locate problems, you should keep records again. We have, after all, taught you a method for analyzing your behavior. You must utilize it to cope with any regression.

It helps to anticipate situations that may bring about regression. Any substantive change in your life can produce one—a new child, a new job, a vacation, an illness—and you ought to try to predict the attendant problems and work out solutions. Awhile ago, for example, a former patient came by and said, "I'm going to have a baby. Will you help me figure out how that's going to change my life? In terms of weight. Once the baby arrives."

We said, "How do *you* think it may change?" And she said, "First, it means that at two in the morning I'm going to have to be awake. Uh oh. What am I going to do at two o'clock in the morning when I'm feeding the baby and I want something to eat." And she began spewing out all her own questions and answers from there.

Another woman and her teen-age son had successfully completed the program together. But now the boy was in the hospital following knee surgery and was due home, in a cast, any day. The woman visited us and said, "People are going to stop by and they're going to bring food because they think that invalids need food. Terrific. That's just what he needs when he can't move, can't get an ounce of activity: food. Just what I need too. What do I do?"

"Talk to the friends in advance," one of us said. "To the ones who are likely to bring food. Tell them, 'Look, both he and I don't really need food. You know we both have a weight problem. So if you're going to bring things, bring puzzles, bring books.' And prepare a list of books you want in case they ask."

When making a major change, consider keeping records even before the scale indicates weight gain. Don't say, "I'll wait for this hectic craziness to die down." Instead, take the view that the day you start a new job might be a good time to simultaneously start records, just to see where the new forces are at work. Perhaps those forces won't produce any extra pounds, but why not be cautious? Admit to yourself at such times: "The new habits I've built may not carry me through this unique circumstance. This is different from anything I've ever encountered before."

Sometimes you may make changes in your life and not think it possible for them to exert any influence on your weight. And abruptly, the scale shows there's a gain and you have no idea why. Again, get out the records. The findings can surprise you, as they did one woman who discovered the reason she'd gained a pound a month for six months was because she'd moved from a two-story house to a two-room apartment. Not only was she getting less activity without stairs to climb, but where once she had been in the habit of spending a lot of time upstairs, now she was much closer to the refrigerator and cupboard and had gotten back into the habit of mindless eating. Moreover, she was nibbling at high-calorie foods she never used to keep around; a steady stream of visitors had been by to see her new place and she'd been storing cakes, cookies, and nuts for them. Her activity patterns, her eating behavior, and her storage habits had all changed.

The message is: Don't panic. Just sit down and spend a couple of hours really thinking back over the program. We sometimes advise people with maintenance problems to make up a list of techniques that helped bring about their weight loss. And often someone will come up with a list of twenty, thirty, thirty-five items. And then look at the list and say, "Hey, here are four key things I'm not doing anymore."

You are capable, really, of being your own detective. Capable of asking yourself questions, of using the tools for maintenance we've provided, of figuring out why you've slipped. The controls may go off momentarily, but that doesn't mean they have to go off forever. Or that to start coping with the problem you have to wait until Monday. If your old habits return for five minutes, next week is not the time to bring them back under control. The most sensible time, the best time, is—exactly—now, right now.

PART 5

Special
Section

CHAPTER
13

Tools for
Maintenance:
A Program
to Live By

TO HELP YOU MAINTAIN YOUR NEW WEIGHT WE HAVE
prepared the following series of checklists and charts.
These will give you the means to: identify and deal
with events that can alter life-style, plan for special
events, make periodic review and self-evaluation of
your habits. These tools for maintenance include a
calorie guide to the menus that have recently become so much a part of America's life on the run;
our fast-food calorie counter will help you enjoy—
and, at the same time cope with—McDonald's, Burger
King, Arthur Treacher's, Burger Chef, Colonel Sanders'
Kentucky Fried Chicken, Long John Silver's, White
Castle, Pizza Hut, Taco Bell and more.

A first step in maintenance, particularly critical if
you find yourself gaining weight, is to review the

techniques that helped you lose pounds in the first place. There are, for starters, the general techniques we offer throughout our program as options for you to choose among. Then there are those techniques that have worked best for you. We recommend that you review both regularly. Here, now, is a list of general techniques for your use. And following that, as a model, is a sample list one of our patients drew up of techniques that worked best for him. Draw up your own, periodically look through it, and ask yourself questions. For example, if teaching yourself to eat more slowly was very helpful in your weight loss, ask yourself:

1. Am I still eating slowly?
2. If not, when did I stop?
3. Was eating slowly helpful?
4. How do I get started again?

GENERAL TECHNIQUES

- Each day keep records of all food eaten
- At home limit all food intake to one specific place
- Rearrange food supplies—adjust packaging and storage habits
- Preplan food intake for each day
- Write down in advance food you plan to eat
- Set up a time schedule each day for meals and snacks
- Make a deliberate decision to eat, don't eat absent-mindedly
- Keep weekly graphs of weight changes and behavior changes
- Regard behavior changes as more important in the long run than immediate weight changes
- Avoid distracting activities while eating

- Be seated while eating
- Do not drop to zero your frequency of eating pre-ferred foods
- Plan in advance for preferred foods
- Keep food out of all rooms other than kitchen and pantry
- Make sure higher caloric foods are not readily available, but require some preparation
- Prepare or take snacks to the table in small quanti-ties
- Have children and spouse prepare their own snacks
- Keep lower caloric foods more available and more visible than higher caloric foods
- Develop a tolerance for hunger by thinking of it more as a positive feeling
- Ask family and friends not to use food for gifts or rewards
- Change your route if a particular store or vending machine you regularly pass by presents a prob-lem

For Meals and Snacks

Plan a short delay before starting to eat

Swallow food before adding more to utensils

Plan a series of brief delays during meals and snacks by:

1. putting down utensils
2. sipping a beverage
3. using a napkin more frequently
4. conversation

Keep extra food away from the table, keep platters in the kitchen

When food platters are on the table, move them away from you

Use measuring spoons and cups to serve

Eat preferred food first

Always leave at least a small amount of food on
  your plate

Clear the table immediately after each course; if
  this is not possible, remove or move your own
  plate

Cover your plate with your napkin as a signal the
  meal has ended

Have someone else remove, store, or throw away
  leftovers if these are a problem

Techniques Useful at Parties and in Restaurants

Look over the entire array of food before beginning
  to eat at a buffet

Sit at a distance from your favorite snack foods

Inquire of the host or hostess what will be served

If you are the host or hostess, give away leftover
  party food

Avoid a long period of deprivation prior to a party
  or eating at a restaurant

Make special requests for combinations and dele-
  tions

Techniques to Be Used between Ingestions

Have a list of activities you can substitute for
  eating at times when you are hungry but have
  not predetermined that you can eat.

Decrease frequency of food shopping

Prepare a complete shopping list

Shop when not hungry

Reduce your purchases of problem foods

Throw out or give away clothes as they become too
  large

Arrange home activities so that your eating place is
  entered infrequently

Physical Activity

Park your car farther away from your destination

Get on or off the bus a few blocks from your stop

Use recreational facilities and opportunities available to you

Replan everyday activities so that more energy is expended

Use a distant rather than a near telephone or bathroom at home

Use the stairs when possible

Miscellaneous

Change self-instruction. For example: "I don't have to eat this now; if I'm hungry later, I can have something to eat."

Be selective and picky about what is eaten

Learn to appreciate the sensory aspects of food

Learn to refuse food effectively and gracefully when pressured

Set realistic goals for vacations and special occasions

Reevaluate your priorities

Reevaluate your life-style

PERSONAL TECHNIQUES

The following is the sample list of changes that worked for one of our patients:

1. Keeping food records
2. Only eating when truly hungry
3. Going to restaurants for my favorite, favorite foods instead of keeping them in the house where they are too tempting
4. "Banking" calories in advance to allow for extra calories for special occasions

5. Treating myself at least once a week to a favorite food
6. Having regularly scheduled weigh-ins at home
7. Using stairs instead of elevators
8. Making meals events when possible, i.e., candlelight, cloth napkins, etc.
9. Not depriving myself of "junk" food
10. Eating real foods, not diet stuff
11. Scheduling snacks to be available when hunger comes
12. Planning interesting activities to be used at periods of hunger
13. Averaging calories weekly and recording the average (as opposed to daily averages)
14. Recognizing the situations that cause me to eat
15. Allowing myself some old habits that weren't so bad after all
16. Going to the grocery store every few *days* instead of every few *weeks*
17. Always grocery shopping from lists and not choosing things impulsively
18. Avoiding grocery aisles that stock food not on my list
19. Eating on a relatively regular time schedule
20. Sleeping on a relatively regular time schedule
21. Rewarding myself with new clothes instead of food on events such as birthdays, anniversaries
22. Carrying a calorie book
23. Walking to work
24. Adding variety on a regular basis
25. Preplanning—creating combination meals and snacks that contain approximately the right amount of calories

PLANNING FOR SPECIAL EVENTS

When maintaining your new weight, just as in losing weight, special events, such as vacations and family reunions, need not be avoided or feared. But they should be planned for in advance

Ask yourself the following questions:
1. Have I been there before (or ever experienced anything similar)?
2. Did I gain weight?
3. How much?
4. What factors were most responsible for the weight gain? Examples: free food, parties, lack of exercise, being cooped up with mother for a week, etc.
5. How did I handle those things then?
6. How could I go about handling them more reasonably this time?
7. Is it unreasonable to expect not to gain some weight in a situation like that?
8. What would be a reasonable expectation of weight gain?

It is a good idea to write out your answer to each question. Keep your answers as a permanent part of a personal weight-control file to be referred to in the future.

LIFE-STYLE CHANGES

As you clearly know by now, changes in your life can have an effect on your eating habits and weight. It is

critical, thus, to pay particular attention to your
eating and activity habits when confronted with a
major life-style change. And it is also important at
such times when you may be confused as to why you
have gained weight to look back and try to determine
if any life-style changes may have been responsible.
The following list represents some of the changes you
should pay particular attention to:

My husband and I are splitting up.

My wife died.

I'm pregnant.

My husband had a heart attack.

My mother is moving in with us.

I just got laid off from work.

I just retired from work.

I became engaged and am getting married in three
    months.

I got a new boss whom I can't get along with.

My best friend moved away.

My daughter just started dating.

My husband is working longer hours.

I just can't get along with my children.

I've got to be in the hospital for two weeks.

I was just promoted to a desk job.

My wife started her own business.

I got a part-time job.

We've decided to adopt a child.

My husband wants to have more children.

My boy started acting up in school.

My kids are all in school now.

I've lost my interest in sex.

We're having another family reunion.

We've lost a lot of money in the stock market.

We just inherited a large sum of money.

My daughter just got married, and they'll be living with us.

We're moving to an apartment in the city.

My daughter's going to college.

My son entered the Army.

My husband and I are getting back together.

I just changed jobs.

My wife and I are arguing more.

I'm responsible for more people at work now.

My wife is going back to work.

I have to work at night this month.

I have to be out-of-town more for my work.

I broke my leg.

I found out I'm diabetic.

We're going to Europe for two weeks.

I'm being audited by the IRS.

I had a fight with one of my friends.

I was elected president of my garden club.

My husband's parents haven't invited us over for a long time.

I'm teaching Sunday school.

My dog was run over by a car.

My cellar was flooded.

My kitchen is being remodeled.

We were snowbound for two days.

This heat wave has lasted for a week.

My kids are home for a two-week vacation.

I'm in charge of food for the county fair.

ASSESSMENT AND EVALUATION

When losing weight, it is essential to be aware of the details of your eating behavior. This is an essential part of maintenance too. We suggest, therefore, that you regularly review your eating habits, perhaps once every four to six weeks. First, go back to your old methods of record keeping: Fill out food diaries for a week and then complete an analysis form. Next dig out an analysis form that has on it your records from one of the weeks back when you were successfully losing weight. After that, on the new forms provided on the following pages enter in the "Then" column the data from a week when you were losing weight in the past. Enter the corresponding data for the current week in the "Now" column. This will permit you to see the exact nature of your eating habits and how they have changed. It will also pinpoint areas that may be in need of new, careful attention.

Upon filling out all the "then and now" forms on the following pages, turn to the final maintenance-assessment form. This one is for the purpose of self-evaluation. The instructions are simple: In the space marked "Eating-Habit Changes" write down any of the differences you have noticed when comparing your eating habits "then" and your eating habits "now." In the space marked "Changes in Life-style" note any life-style shifts you feel may have caused changes in your eating habits or in your physical-activity patterns. If these changes have caused weight gain, or seem likely to, write down, under "Necessary Steps," what you plan to do about them. Also review your lists of general techniques and personal techniques, and note under "Necessary Steps" any of those you feel require renewed attention.

BURNING UP CALORIES THROUGH ACTIVITY
(Amount varies according to individual)

Activity	Per Hour	15 Minutes	Five Minutes
	Approximate calories burned:		
Walking (2 miles per hour)	200	50	17
(5 miles per hour)	650	162	54
Light Gardening	240	60	20
Carpentry	230	57	19
Light housework	180	45	15
Driving an automobile	140	35	12
House painting	210	52	17
Heavy gardening (digging)	500	125	42
Bicycling (slow)	300	75	25
(strenuous)	600	150	50
Swimming (leisurely)	400	100	33
(rapid)	800	200	67
Golf	250	62	21
Tennis (singles)	450	112	37
(doubles)	350	87	29
Skiing (downhill)	450	112	37
(cross-country)	1200	300	100
Rowing (slow)	400	100	33
(fast)	800	200	67
Handball	550	137	46
Bowling	250	62	21
Squash	550	137	46
Fishing	150	37	12
Fast Dancing	600	150	50
Motorcycling	150	37	12
Jogging	600	150	50
Badminton	350	87	29

MAINTENANCE ASSESSMENT

I. Time of Eating   THEN (date)_____

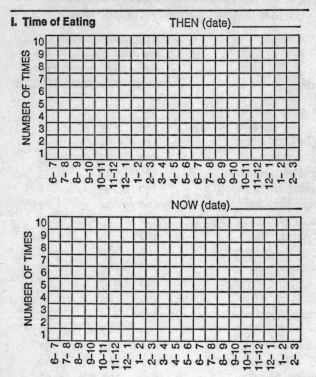

NOW (date)_____

II. Duration of Eating	**MEALS**		**SNACKS**	
	THEN	NOW	THEN	NOW
0–4 Minutes				
5–10 Minutes				
11–20 Minutes				
Over 20 Minutes				

III. Place of Eating	MEALS		SNACKS	
	THEN	NOW	THEN	NOW
Kitchen				
Dining Room				
Living Room				
Bedroom				
Den				
Car				
Bus, Train				
Walking				
Office				
Restaurant				
Friend's Home				
Other				

IV. Physical Position				
Standing				
Sitting				
Lying Down				

V. Alone or With Whom				
Alone				
Spouse				
Family				
Friends				
Business Associates				
Strangers				
Other				

MAINTENANCE ASSESSMENT (cont'd)

	MEALS		SNACKS	
VI. Associated Activity	THEN	NOW	THEN	NOW
Eating Only				
Talking				
Reading				
Radio, Music				
Television				
Cooking				
Other				
VII. Mood				
Neutral				
Content				
Happy				
Tense				
Depressed				
Angry				
Bored				
Fatigued				
Rushed				
VIII. Degree of Hunger				
0–2 (None to Mild)				
3–5 (Mild to Extreme)				
IX. Type of Food				
Alcohol				
Baked Goods				
Cake, Cookies,				
Crackers, etc.				
Candy				
Cheese				
Ice Cream, Sherbet				
Jam				
Jello				

Type of Food (cont'd)	MEALS		SNACKS	
	THEN	NOW	THEN	NOW
Nuts				
Peanut Butter				
Potato Chips, etc.				
Pretzels				
Sodas				
Diet				
Regular				
Sugar				
Coffee-mate				
Bread, Rolls				
Butter, Margarine				
Cereal				
Condiments				
Eggs				
Fish				
Fruit				
Juice				
Mayonnaise				
Meat				
Milk				
Whole				
Skim				
Pasta Products				
Pizza				
Potatoes				
Poultry				
Salads				
Salad Dressing				
Soups				
Syrups, Sauces				
Vegetables				
Waffles, Pancakes				
Yogurt, Cottage Ch.				

MAINTENANCE ASSESSMENT

Weekly Caloric Intake

THEN _____

NOW _____

Changes in Life-style (see Instructions)

_____

_____

_____

_____

_____

_____

_____

_____

_____

_____

_____

_____

_____

_____

_____

Eating-Habit Changes (see instructions)

_____

_____

_____

_____

_____

_____

_____

_____

_____

_____

_____

Necessary Steps

_____

_____

_____

_____

_____

_____

The Fast-Food
Calorie Counter

Each day fast-food chains sell millions of meals and snacks to Americans. And yet we find that even people who are well-informed about calories are generally unable to estimate or find out the caloric content of what they eat in fast-food restaurants. The following list will help fill this information gap.

It is important to know the calories in what you eat at the fast-food restaurants. And it is critical, too, to understand the impact these places have upon your overall eating behavior. Fast rates of eating, inability to control portion size, absence of utensils and limited food selections lead to habitual rapid ingestion with a low level of food awareness. You must be particularly careful, then, in fast-food restaurants, to utilize those eating techniques that have helped you take off—and keep off—weight you don't want.

ARTHUR TREACHER'S   CALORIES
Chips (serving) 274
Coleslaw 122
Fish (per piece) 172

BASKIN-ROBBINS
One Scoop:
Ice Creams, all flavors .... between
133 and 148
Sherbets and Ices 139

BURGER CHEF
Big Shef 535
French Fries 240
Hamburger 250
Shake, Chocolate 310
Super Shef 530

BURGER KING
Cheeseburger 305
French Fries 220
Hamburger 230
Hamburger, Double 325
Shake, Chocolate 365
Whopper 630
Whopper Junior 285

COLONEL SANDERS'
KENTUCKY FRIED CHICKEN
Dinner (Fried Chicken, Mashed Potatoes,
Coleslaw, Rolls):
2-Piece Dinner—Original 595
Crispy 665
3-Piece Dinner—Original 980
Crispy 1070

DAIRY QUEEN/BRAZIER   CALORIES

"Bosn's Mate" Fish Sandwich	340
"Brazier"	250
"Brazier" Barbeque	280
"Brazier" Cheeseburger	310
"Brazier" Chili Dog	330
"Brazier" Dog	270
"Brazier" French Fries	200
"Brazier" Onion Rings	300
Big "Brazier"	510
Big "Brazier" Cheeseburger	600
Big "Brazier" Deluxe	540
Super "Brazier" Chili Dog	570
Super "Brazier" Dog	500
Super "Brazier"/The "Half Pounder"	850

Ice Creams

Banana Split	580
"Buster Bar"*	390
"Dairy Queen" Cones*:	
Small	110
Medium	230
Large	340
"Dairy Queen" Dipped Cones*:	
Small	160
Medium	310
Large	450
"Dairy Queen" Malts*:	
Small	400
Medium	580
Large	830

* All other flavors have fewer calories than chocolate; figures for chocolate given, since it's the most popular flavor.

"Dairy Queen" Sundaes*:	CALORIES
Small	190
Medium	300
Large	430
"Dilly Bar"*	240
"DQ" Sandwich*	190
Hot fudge "Brownie Delight" sundae	580
Pârfait	460

DUNKIN DONUTS

Donuts and Cake, including Chocolate Cake (includes rings, sticks, crullers)	240
Donuts, Yeast Raised (add 5–10 calories for glaze)	160
Fancies (includes coffee rolls, Danish, etc.)	215
Munchkins, Yeast Raised	26
Cake, including Chocolate Cake	66

(Add 40–50 calories per Donut for filling and topping combined; add 10–15 calories per Munchkin for filling and topping combined. Figures are approximations.)

GINO'S

Apple Pie	198
Cheeseburger	336
Coke (regular)	117
Coke (giant)	181
Dinner Roll	51
Fry (regular)	195
Fry (giant)	274
Hamburger	289
Kentucky Fried Chicken (1 piece)	290
Orange (regular)	140
Orange (giant)	217

* All other flavors have fewer calories than chocolate; figures for chocolate given, since it's the most popular flavor.

CALORIES

Root Beer (regular)	122
Root Beer (giant)	190
Shake, Vanilla (regular)	338
Shake, Vanilla (giant)	524
Sirloiner	514
Sirloiner (Cheese)	609

HOWARD JOHNSON'S

Baked Beans*	150
Croquettes (Chicken)*	192.9
Croquettes (Shrimp)*	171.7
Haddock au Gratin*	114.6
Ice Cream (Chocolate)*	261
Ice Cream (Vanilla)*	247
Macaroni and Cheese**	191
Meat Balls*	230
Meat Loaf*	243
Salisbury Steak*	214
Sherbet*	138
Toastees (Blueberry)	341
Toastees (Cinnamon Raisin)	372
Toastees (Corn)	315
Toastees (Orange)	398
Toastees (Pound Cake)	391

LONG JOHN SILVER'S

Fish & Chips, Coleslaw

2-Piece Dinner	955
3-Piece Dinner	1190

* Basic Serving 100 gm. Servings sometimes vary from the list; each franchise can explain how much.
** Serving usually 200 gm., or double the calorie count.

MCDONALD'S   CALORIES

Apple Pie 265
Big Mac 557
Cheeseburger 309
Egg McMuffin 312
Fillet-O-Fish 406
French Fries 215
Hamburger 249
Hamburger, Double 350
Hot Cakes with butter 272
Muffin 136
Pork Sausage 235
¼ Pounder 414
¼ Pounder with Cheese 521
Scrambled Eggs 175
Shake, Chocolate 317
Shake, Strawberry 315
Shake, Vanilla 322

PIZZA HUT

½ of 13-Inch Cheese Pizza—Thick Crust 900
                      Thin Crust 850
½ of 15-Inch Cheese Pizza—Thick Crust 1200
                      Thin Crust 1150

½ of 10-Inch (Thin Crust)
        Beef 488
        Cheese 436
        Pepperoni 459
        Pork 466
        Supreme 475

RUSTLER STEAK HOUSE

Baked Potato 231
Dressing (Blue Cheese) 151

CALORIES

Dressing (French)	122
Dressing (Italian)	166
Dressing (Thousand Island)	150
Jello, Cherry	75
Margarine Potato	215
Pickles	2
Potato Chips	82
Pudding, Chocolate	144
Roll (Butter)	40
Roll (Margarine)	53
Roll (Rustler)	120
Roll (Twisted)	182
Rib Eye	369
Rustler's (Strip)	1086
Salad	13
Steak (Chopped) 4 oz.	327
Steak (Chopped) 8 oz.	653
T-Bone	1532

TACO-BELL

Beans (Whipped) Burito	345
Bell Burger	243
Enchirito	391
Frejoles	231
Taco	146
Tostado	206

WHITE CASTLE

Cheeseburger	198
Fish Sandwich	200
French Fries	219
Hamburger	165
Milk Shake	213
Onion Rings	341

About the Authors

HENRY A. JORDAN, M.D., is co-director of the Institute for Behavioral Education, King of Prussia, Pennsylvania, and an Associate Clinical Professor of Psychiatry at the School of Medicine of the University of Pennsylvania.

LEONARD S. LEVITZ, Ph.D., is co-director of the Institute for Behavioral Education, King of Prussia, Pennsylvania, and an Assistant Clinical Professor of Psychology in Psychiatry, School of Medicine, University of Pennsylvania.

GORDON M. KIMBRELL, Ph.D., is Director of the Center for Effective Living, Granville, Ohio, and Associate Professor of Psychology at Dennison College.

STEVE GELMAN, formerly Articles Editor of *Life* Magazine, is a free-lance writer and editor for, among others, Time-Life Books and the Time Inc. Magazine Development Group. He has written for numerous magazines, including *Life*, *Esquire* and *New York*, and has been author of—and/or editor-collaborator on—several books.

Index